ANXIETY

How to Overcoming Depression, Shyness and Gain Better Self Social Confidence

(Use Self-hypnosis and Affirmations for Stress Relief)

Ellen Wallace

Published by Kevin Dennis

© **Ellen Wallace**

All Rights Reserved

Anxiety in Relationships: How to Overcoming Depression, Shyness and Gain Better Self Social Confidence (Use Self-hypnosis and Affirmations for Stress Relief)

ISBN 978-1-989920-41-1

Legal & Disclaimer

The information contained in this book is not designed to replace or take the place of any form of medicine or professional medical advice. The information in this book has been provided for educational and entertainment purposes only.

The information contained in this book has been compiled from sources deemed reliable, and it is accurate to the best of the Author's knowledge; however, the Author cannot guarantee its accuracy and validity and cannot be held liable for any errors or omissions. Changes are periodically made to this book. You must consult your doctor or get professional medical advice before using any of the suggested remedies, techniques, or information in this book.

Upon using the information contained in this book, you agree to hold harmless the Author from and against any damages, costs, and expenses, including any legal fees potentially resulting from the application of any of the information provided by this guide. This disclaimer applies to any damages or injury caused by the use and application, whether directly or indirectly, of any advice or information presented, whether for breach of contract, tort, negligence, personal injury, criminal intent, or under any other cause of action.

You agree to accept all risks of using the information presented inside this book. You need to consult a professional medical practitioner in order to ensure you are both able and healthy enough to participate in this program.

Table of Contents

Introduction

This book contains proven steps and strategies on how to conquer your fears when taking exams.

Similarly, the book expounds on key techniques to help you develop the right attitude, particularly when it comes to preparing for exams. As it were, getting ready to take exams is something most students dread. In most cases, however, these apprehensions come about as a product of fears of failure, unrealistic expectations, bad study habits, and sheer lack of preparation. This book will help you in combatting these things and aid you in forming a holistic approach to taking exams.

Thanks again for downloading this book, I hope you enjoy it!

Chapter 1: What Causes Mental Clutter?

Mental clutter is an easy phrase to describe the vastness of your thoughts, memories, and experiences. Every aspect of your daily life gets stored in your brain, and in such a small space, there is bound to be clutter. While it isn't known exactly why or how we can remember so many things, what we do know is that there is certainly a capacity at which we overload ourselves, and our overall function suffers from it.

Mental clutter is often synonymous with emotional baggage. We often let episodes from our past give weight and value to our present. For example, if you failed an important task at work, and you let it define you, an air of doubt is cast over your current work and ability.

Carrying on poor relationships is a big driver of mental clutter. Ideally, we would all like to say that we are in supportive, coexisting relationships. In reality, we all have relationships that are emotionally draining, at best. Think of that friend who always needs something, or always has something heavy weighing on them. Doesn't some of that negativity get transferred to you?

Is your home or work situation conducive to great emotions? Is your partner in crime really dedicated to you, or is the relationship forced? We often settle for relationships that are less than supportive for the sake of not being alone. At work, you may be surrounded by people who really want to see you fail, even if they seem supportive on the surface.

It is important to recognize these flaws in relationships so you may avoid the obvious pitfalls. It will always be necessary to carry on relationships that don't exactly suit you, but the goal is to navigate them in a way that benefits you. There will always be a bit of negativity, but if you make the conscious decision to avoid it, your emotional conscience will be clear, and your degree of mental clutter will be low.

You have the right to avoid drama in your life. We all know one person in our lives who always has something bad going on, or gets caught up in anything and everything bad. Their sister is having a fight with her husband, and it is making them sad today. They need to make sure their grown children are getting off to work, and their husband's sister-in-law's friend had a death in the family, and suddenly get wrapped up in that. The downward spiral that ensues is inevitable. If you don't feel you know someone like that, take a look at yourself. This is probably you!

Getting involved in this drama is against your better judgment, and you know it. The trick is separating yourself from situations that bring you down. Yes, it is conducive to a good friend to be there for friends when bad things are happening. However, it is another situation entirely to engross yourself and get caught up in that negative energy. Oftentimes, you are only fueling that negativity when you choose to be part of it.

Very simply, mental clutter is anything that gets in the way of your focus at any given moment. That is, if you are thinking of other things, you are not wholly focused on whatever is going on in the here and now. This can certainly be emotional, as described above, but can be very simple things in life that bog you down as well. This can manifest itself in a number of ways.

We often see multitasking as a great thing, a real talking point on your resume. Being able to juggle many things at once is a valuable skill sought by most employers. This has also become insidious in our daily life. The ability to work, care for a family, make dinner and have a side hustle is considered the norm these days.

The reality is, if your mind is forced to focus attention on all of these things at once, it is not giving its undivided attention on any one thing. This is a real jack-of-all-trades, master-of-none kind of moment. What are you really gaining from doing so many things if you aren't doing any of them as well as you could? Think of the potential you could harness if you could just focus on one thing. Wouldn't you really knock it out of the park if all your attention was dedicated to something?

Mental clutter manifests itself outside as well. Environmental clutter is both a symptom of mental clutter and a cause of it. That is, what you surround yourself with can affect your mood and your ability to think straight.

Consider the state of your home or office space for a moment? Is it conducive to clear thinking? Are your spaces clear of unneeded items, paperwork, and junk? Does everything have a space? Are there things out of place? All of these things unwittingly tax the mind. Your brain likes order, and when things are out of place, the mind tries to make sense of it. The mind will begin to wander, thinking about the dishes in the sink, the sock on the floor, the laundry pile, and putting things away.

Meanwhile, really productive, happy, exciting thoughts are pushed to the corner because the brain is already exhausted. It is really difficult to brainstorm for your business or have a candid moment when your brain is otherwise preoccupied. Take a look at your surroundings and assess whether or not it looks like a blank slate for thought, or if it looks like a to-do list.

Mental clutter is unavoidable all the time, but with the help of the ideas interwoven in this book, it is possible to eliminate and avoid adding new clutter in your daily life. Good navigation will allow your mind to focus on the task at hand, and really tap in to what is important and valuable in your life. Allowing this action is conducive to living your best life.

How Minds Get Cluttered

So how do our brains get cluttered? Well, everyone has clutter accumulated in their minds. We will tackle ways to prevent cluttering, and we will have a look into one of the most common ways to break the clutter – living a simpler life.

As we already stated, the best way to declutter your mind is to be informed on why your brain is cluttered in the first place. In other words, one of the main reasons people have so much negative energy is because they lack knowledge regarding brain clutter. The majority of the population does not know what clutter is and explains it as something totally different, blaming either the context, others, or themselves.

The mechanism that clutters our mind is fueled by our uncertainty and social conventions. We live in a society that praises individualism, success, strength, and determination.

When we face obstacles in achieving those, clutter begins to form. But is there a way to prevent it from happening in the first place?

There is good news and bad news. The good news is, being self-aware and having a more relaxed view on things can definitely prevent the start of the cluttering process. The bad news is, staying positive and relaxed, without stress about small and insignificant things is virtually impossible nowadays.

There is no way we could pass through life without interacting with what the present time holds. Unless we choose from the start to isolate ourselves from all that is human and social, becoming monks or taking the ascetic road, it is obvious that we have to deal with the challenges and not run away from them.

Going even further with the comparison, a body that wants to prevent illness and disease cannot simply run away from pathogens, and isolate itself from any possible harm. That would achieve the opposite results: our immune system would not be formed; we would become weak and more exposed to getting sick. The same can be applied to our mind. It is never a solution to stay away, and even if some precautions should be taken, living life to the full is definitely the way to go about it. What if all of us choose to get away, and run from each other and isolate ourselves? Hard to imagine, isn't it?

We all know that when falling in love, for example, there is a great deal of risk that love will eventually cause suffering. But that never stopped anyone from searching for love. We know the price, and we are happily ready to pay it. It is part of our existence, so we don't even question it.

The same applies to our mind and the risk of cluttering. Preventing the formation of such clutter is a definite possibility, but acting upon what our immense, complex, and beautiful mind reveals is not debatable. We cannot just put half of our brain on pause. It wouldn't be fair; it wouldn't benefit anyone. So, we can only rely on staying on top of things, being informed and accessing the knowledge that could prevent the creeping in of clutter while at the same time enjoy the huge array of possibilities that are derived from it.

Chapter 2: Mindful Breathing

"Breathing in, I calm body and mind. Breathing out, I smile.

Dwelling in the present moment, I know this is the only moment.

~ Thich Nhất Hạnh

Do you remember your last breath? I bet you're aware of the one you just took after reading that question. The average person takes over 20,000 breaths a day, and unless our attention is drawn to our breathing for some reason, we aren't aware of most of those breaths. Although it's essential for our survival, breathing isn't something we give much thought to.

Breathing is important for two reasons: it supplies our bodies and organs with the oxygen necessary for survival, and it rids our bodies of waste products. Oxygen is essential for our brains, nerves, glands, and internal organs. Without it, we would die within minutes. If the brain is deprived

12

of oxygen, it can damage other organs and systems in our bodies. Lack of oxygen is a major cause of heart disease, strokes, and cancer.

We are mostly unconscious of our breathing, and therefore, we don't recognize when we're breathing improperly. In fact, you may not realize there is a proper and improper way to breath. Is there something more than just sucking in air and releasing it? Although breathing is managed in the unconscious, at any moment, we can take over and consciously change how we breathe. Our modern lifestyles make conscious breathing more important than you can imagine.

Chapter 3: Causes Of Stress, Dangers And When To Make Extreme Change.

Like anything in life, there are varying degrees and levels of our experiences. Stress is no different. It may turn up in our lives in various situations. Something as simple as having a job interview for example. Or you may be a student, studying long hours in order to master a profession, or a parent who works overtime to provide for their children. Regardless of the situation, stress comes and goes. Sometimes the best things in life however, demand the sacrifice of happiness as payment. In cases like this, stress may push us to perform. Often, professional athletes utilize stress in order to achieve phenomenal results. This is the kind of daily stress which is quite manageable, and can even be used to your advantage. Some sacrifice or endurance to stress is sometimes necessary.

But you have to be careful not to give or sacrifice too much. Like the isolated mother or father who never go out, and have no friends who may in turn burden their children with their loneliness. Or the tired partner who floats to work and home, lifeless like a zombie who could become useless at both the workplace and at home. Or the young student, unable to focus, can become overwhelmed with life.

At the extreme, you hear stories in the news of people who work to exhaustion and the hopeless who resort to killing themselves.

We need to clearly identify the difference between simple daily life stresses and situations which could potentially be dangerous. Too much stress - or what is known as extreme stress can cause serious illness or even potentially be life threatening.

Sometimes we know deep down that a life change has to be made, but we just don't take action. We keep telling ourselves that things will get better or really, things aren't as bad as we make them out to be. But you need to ask yourself - will things really get better?

Take for example an abusive or violent relationship. The kind of stress a situation such as this causes should not have to be endured. The same goes for a boss or co-worker in your place of employment, that might be verbally abusing you or constantly putting you down. Or possible financial debt that could lead to you losing your house or to a messy divorce. These kinds of situations will put you under extreme stress and the outcome will always be detrimental to your physical and mental health. If you are in any situations like this and there's only one thing that you can take away from this book; then it should be this - Walk away! Don't stay in the abusive relationship or the never-ending hopeless loop. Or work towards improving your finances. No form of stress management will help you with these kinds of problems. The only cure is to distance yourself from - or fix the situation!

If you believe that you are in a situation that may feel hopeless, then it is best to make a change as soon as possible.

Chapter 4: Physical Health And Anxiety

"It all begins with you. If you do not care for your own self, you will not be strong enough to take care of anything in life" - Leon Brown

Relation of Physical and Mental health

Mind and body should not be thought of as separate from one another. They are both responsible for the proper functioning of a human being. If one health is declining, then there is definitely going to be an effect on the other.

People suffering from distress are 32% more likely to die from cancer than those who don't have self-induced distress about the disease. ("Physical health and mental health", 2019)[5]. Schizophrenia is also a mental disorder that doubles the risk of heart disease and increases the risk of respiratory disease by three times. Depression has been associated directly to heart problems.

This chapter would help in the realization that physical health should also be taken care of if you suffer from mental health issues.

Anxiety Disorders

There is not one identifiable cause of anxiety which will pinpoint its exact origin. However, there are some factors that are identified by researchers of mental health. According to them, these circumstances make us prone to anxiety disorders.

Anxiety disorders are more often than not appear to run in families. Although, there is no proof that genetic factors are involved. It may just be that environmental factors surrounding that particular household that are the cause.

Personality is the major factor in determining how we perceive everyday life and our behavior to our environment. More often, introverts are prone to anxiety than extroverts. Some people are perfectionists and some like to just get things done. Generally, low self-esteem arises from overthinking and poor coping mechanisms. All these things are mostly found in people who suffer from depression.

Neurotransmitters' lack or excess is also directly related to anxiety. Imbalance in them causes the anxiety-producing pathways to react more than normal.

Some illnesses such as long term heart disease or diabetes are sometimes the cause of an anxiety disorder. It might not be illness itself but a person's reaction to it. A feeling of helplessness can quickly bring on depression. If this is not identified and dealt with, then it will soon develop into anxiety.

Some hormonal gland problems have been directly linked to causing stress and anxiety.

Caffeine can make anxiety symptoms worse. Alcohols and drugs are also known to enhance the anxiety of the user.

Sometimes, a single event can turn it upside down for you. The occurrence of a horrible event may have had caused huge distress upon a person. Its consequences could be detrimental to a person's mental health. For example, abuse, the death of a loved one, a relationship cut-off, hectic jobs, etc. are some common events that have a huge impact on a person. It could also lead to developing severe anxiety.

Lifestyle Factors Affecting Both Types of Health

Here are some of the things you can do that would help in improving both your mental and physical health.

Diet

Ever heard the phrase "you are what you eat." It is true even though we eat every day, it's a common activity and we don't really pay attention to it, except those who are health freaks. It is a good thing to be concerned about what you are eating. Eating is one of the most important things needed for survival after all.

A good healthy diet will keep us healthy and the opposite will bring on a number of problems that make themselves appear over time. A healthy diet of fats, proteins, vitamins, minerals, and carbohydrates is essential to nutrition. The diet we intake can influence our physical health and it becomes pretty apparent to us over time. What we eat can directly influence mental health disorders such as Alzheimer's and depression.

Exercise

Any kind of positive physical activity is very important for our physical health. What we don't pay attention to is how it is necessary for our mental health as well. It is proven by research that doing exercise will release endorphins in the brain.They are feel-good chemicals that lift the mod. They will increase your awareness and energy. Even just walking for a while has an amazing impact on one's mood.

By physical activity, it means expending energy by movements that involve your muscles. Even just doing normal chores around the house will improve your mental health and you will have a clean house in the end. Exercise is a win-win situation for your body and brain.

Smoking

It is pretty much established that smoking is extremely harmful to your health. The funny thing is most people claim to do it for mental health reasons. They feel like they can effectively reduce their depression and stress through it. But it is only a short term solution and in the long run, its consequences outweigh whatever momentary benefits it presents.

People with depression are more likely to smoke than other people.

Cigarettes contain nicotine. It is a chemical that disrupts and alters chemicals in our brain. People with depression have lower levels of dopamine. Dopamine is responsible for inducing the positive feeling in our brains. Nicotine temporarily increases the production of dopamine. In the long run, it severely affects the natural ability to produce more dopamine in the future. So a person winds up addicted to smoking just because they think it is the answer to their troubles.

Effects of Anxiety on Physical Health

Anxiety has a considerable effect on our physical health not only for short term but also in the long run. If it, unfortunately, goes on for long, a person could develop chronic physical conditions.

When a person starts to get anxious or stressed, the brain sends signals to the body. Our body ends up releasing adrenaline and cortisol. Both of these are stress hormones. They are only good for the body when we are in actual danger, not for everyday life situations.

Some of the negative effects anxiety can have on our body systems involve:

1.Respiratory systems

Hyperventilation is when a person has difficulty breathing. It becomes shallow and rapid. This occurs during anxiety. During this whole process, the body intakes much more oxygen to supply to the brain. They often began gasping for breath as they feel a heightened need for it. Some of its accompanying symptoms are weakness, dizziness, lightheadedness, and the feeling that you are about to faint.

2.Cardiovascular system

As anxiety can change the breathing pattern so directly, it will also affect the heartbeat too. It can cause a change in heart rate and circulation.

This all is to cater for the fight-or-flight response your brain has told your body to do. Your muscles will start getting more oxygen and nutrients because it makes your body think you are in a fight with someone when really you will only be stressed for a test.

Hot flashes can also occur in the body. It happens when our blood vessels narrow, which is called vasoconstriction. Vasoconstriction affects the temperature of the body. After then, the body starts sweating apparently to cool down but then you end up feeling cold.

3.Immune system

All the boost our body gets from anxiety is short-lived and for the long run, it messes up our immune system badly.

People with more serious anxiety disorders tend to get more flu and colds.

4.Digestive system

Cortisol is a stress hormone. It is released during any situation where we are threatened or when under distress. Its function is to block off the processes of the body that are nonessential in a fight-or-flight situation. As digestion is not particularly needed in a threatening situation, it turns that down as well. Adrenaline is the culprit too as it blocks the blood flow and stomach muscles relax. As a result, you feel nausea and lose your appetite. It also causes diarrhea and you feel like your stomach is upset. There is also some research to suggest that depression can cause irritable bowel syndrome.

5.Urinary

So during a fight-or-flight response, it is natural to have an empty bladder. So that it would make us run faster. That is why we tend to get an increased urge to urinate whenever we are anxious or under stress.

Simple Practices for Wellbeing

One of the best things that you can do to practice wellbeing is exercise. Putting your body under stress will reduce the stress off your brain.

You don't have to exercise like everybody else. Any other physical activity will be just as good if not better. You will enjoy it also so overall it will become an activity that you will look forward to and enjoy doing.

There are supplements proven to reduce anxiety and depression. Some of them are

•Lemon balm

•Omega-3 fatty acids

•Ashwagandha

•Green tea

- Valerian

- Kava Kava

Candles are great for aesthetic and lighting up your mood. The scented ones or essential oils will help reduce the feeling of stress and help produce a peaceful effect on your surroundings.

Aromatherapy is the use of scents to make your mood better. Some of the soothing scents are

- Rose

- Sandalwood

- Lavender

High dosage of caffeine can promote anxiety. Especially if you notice signs that after caffeine intake, you get jittery, then consider cutting it out of your life. It can be healthy in moderate amounts. You should test out your threshold for caffeine intake and notice if you experience anxiety more afterward.

Talking about your feelings isn't always easy. Finding an outlet for your feelings and thoughts is a very healthy way to deal with them. One of those outlets is writing. Writing about your feelings and thoughts can help you positively confront them as well as letting them out. Bottling up your feelings is never a healthy thing.

Writing about both negative and positive things in your life is a progressive habit and it will help you grow as a person. By recording negative thoughts, you are facing them in a clearer perspective. By writing positive things, you are being thankful for their existence.

Chewing gum. Believe it or not, it has a number of physical and mental health benefits. People who chewed gum has a greater sense of wellbeing according to a study. They experience lower levels of stress. Chewing gum makes more blood flow to the brain. It produces brain waves that are the same as of those people who are relaxed (Smith, Chaplin & Wadsworth, 2012)[6]. Did you ever observe that whenever something stressful is going on a person tends to chew gum more aggressively? Well, a recent study found that stress relief happens more when gum is chewed more aggressively.

Don't underestimate the power of friendship. Having a good friend is a treasure. Spending time around your loved ones, who are there to support you will give a feeling of belonging. It will help reduce depression. People with few friends are also more likely to suffer from anxiety. Spend time on your relationships. Try connecting with people; however, you are comfortable.

Laughter is good for your health. It relieves stress and tension in your body.

Listen to your favorite tunes.

Having a pet can give you a sense of purpose and keep you active. It will also be a great company. These are all the best ways to combat anxiety.

Learn to stay on top of your schedule. Having things burden up on you will likely cause a lot of stress. Simply don't put off what can be done today for tomorrow.

Keep yourself productively busy, try not to limit yourself by thinking that you are not up to doing certain hobbies. Learn to approach life with an open mind. Having a number of interests and pursuing those staves off anxiety.

If you are in a position to give back to the world, then do so. Simple volunteer work is great if you can do so. Even a smile or thank you counts a lot in the rash world today.

The best thing you can do for your mind is not to overthink. Learn to be in the moment and be mindful as explained in the previous chapter.

Chapter 5: Talk About Your Fears

A problem shared is half solved goes a popular aphorism. Talking to people about your fears is one of the easiest ways to fight and overcome your fears. When you talk to people about what your challenges, fears, dreams and passions; you lift and relieve your overburdened soul, it lightens your heart. It gives you a sense of freedom and breathes some needed confidence into you.There exits bundles of testimonies of how people have overcome one challenge or the other by merely talking about it with people. Talking about your fears systematically melts the fear off your heart, unveils it, and makes it appear ordinary. Talking about your fear gives you makes you overcome solitude and sorrow as it enlivens you and clears your thought.

4.1. Why Should I Talk to People About my Fears?

Talking to people about your fears provides you with an avenue to rub minds with other people. A sense of belonging.

It affords you the opportunity to meet people going through similar situations and challenges with you and shows you that you are not alone.

It gives you the chance to learn pragmatic and practical ways to fight your fears from experienced people who had similar fears, fought and defeated such fears.

It helps you learn how people have climbed through their fears to greatness and glory.

It provides an objective and diverse opinions to your situation which in turn leaves you with many solutions you can pick from.

4.2. Who is in the Best position to talk to?

Right, you cannot just talk to anyone about your passions or fears. Why? Simply because only few people care about you and your dreams. The modern world is such an individualistic one that people care-less about others. People are blind with ego and self-centeredness. There are jesters and dream-killers that would rather than soothe your soul bring you more pain; discourage rather than encourage, laugh and scorn rather than show concern. There are numerous soul-less souls on this planet. However, there are people you cannot hide your true situation from; people you can lean and cry on their shoulders. Who are these people? Your close-friends, family members, lover, and mentor are people that you can open-up to, share your inner feelings, thoughts, struggles, goals and fears with it. They would listen with their hearts, provide succor, make you believe in yourself and dreams and give sincere pieces of advice.

4.3. Consult a Professional

If you are scared or shy to talk to the persons above or you feel that your loved ones have not being objective and sincere in their interpretation of your situation due to their emotional attachment to you(a valid point though), it isadvisable to seek the help of a professional counselor.A professional counselor would critically and objectively observe and dissect your fears, the probable causes and how best to confront it and gain victory over it. You should however try to be as truthful as possible: without any ounce of deceit -- Tell it all. What about my deepest secrets? You can be rest assured that your secrets are safe with a professional, he/she is bound by the law to keep whatever you have discussed as discreet as possible. That is what makes him/her a professional. It is that simple!

It is important to note that the type of fear you nurse in your heart will determine the kind of person(s) to talk about it with. Fears about the future should be discussed with someone who has so much experience about life, most preferably, an aged man/woman (your grandparents), fears relating to starting a business or other business stuffs should be discussed with a leading and successful entrepreneur in the business world, fears about relationship and love should be discussed with happily married people and so on. Never discuss your fears with failures; they have nothing positive to offer you, they would only get things complicated and messier for you.

4.4. Chapter To-Do

Go find the sheet you kept in your diary.

Go through the written fears and identify the most appropriate person(s) to discuss them with.

Book an appointment with them to discuss through your fears.

Note and write the salient idea you got from each person you spoke with

Chapter 6: The Nature Of Anxiety

These situations are charged with the similar emotion: anxiety. When you feel stressed, you feel anxious. Let's take a moment to understand what this complicated feeling really is. Anxiety is a preoccupation with the future. There is an event in the future and you are concerned with it in the present. For students, they are anxious about their grades. So at the present, they are waiting, but the grades which ate not yet given stresses them. They might even be more stressed, not with the grades, but with how their parents may react. For employees, they might be anxious about keeping their jobs. They still have it, but they worry about a time they may be terminated.

Being in the future, the projected events may or may not happen. You may bring an umbrella today because of a weather forecast of 50% chance of rain. But it may or may not rain. Unless a contest is rigged, in a competition, there is no assurance of a 100% chance of winning or losing. Until the very last moment, it can be anybody's game. The closest thing we can describe future events is probabilities. There is a probability of being fired from a job, or hitting the jackpot or getting into an accident. As the term implies, we are talking of things that may or may not probably happen. We can use statistics to create some sense of order, but they are not absolute. You can be 99% sure that it will rain tomorrow but there is still a 1% chance it may not. Prediction and projection are not absolute realities because they are still in a future which has not happened.

Anxiety makes the future thing a present concern. The stress builds up precisely because we feel powerless over a future we cannot control. The future becomes very frightening for some people because they have no handle on it now. Some people are afraid of trying a new exotic food because they haven't tasted it and they worry about its safety. They cannot know unless they actually try it. The loss of control may be traumatic for some people. People work all their lives to gain control over things. Insurance is actually built on trying to mitigate or control a future which has not happened. We exert all measures to gain control over things. The more we can control something, the more assured we will feel. And if we cannot control things, anxiety steps in.

We can also trace anxiety developmentally. We begin life in the womb and it is the most secure place in the world. There is constant nourishment, the environment is warm, and there is a great sense of security. Birthing is the first traumatic experience of being expelled from this Paradise and we are thrust into a hostile world. We cannot have food immediately; we need to cry to be attended to. Our mother is our go-to person, the care provider we seek for security and nourishment. We feel at peace when we are cradled and we are fed from her breasts. But at times, our experience of mothering can also be traumatized. There will be times when she is not around when we need her. Anxiety develops because we feel threatened by the loss of our primary care provider. When she returns, we feel at peace again. When she doesn't, the anxiety deepens. The attachment between mother and child becomes the basis of our capacity to trust and to be independent. A healthy attachment develops if a mother can leave her baby and return to him or her with regularity. The baby is able to be independent and still trusting of his or her mother. Unhealthy attachment occurs if the mother never leaves the baby so the baby never develops independence or there is irregularity in the return. In that case, the baby learns to mistrust the mother because the care is unpredictable. An anxious personality develops. These attachment theories have been developed by psychologists like Sigmund Freud, Mary Ainsworth and John Bowlby. The theories try to explain how attachment develops and how anxiety progresses as a result of the unresolved conflict.

Childhood anxieties are carried over adolescence and throughout our adult lives. Levels of anxiety differ according to the situation and to our personal histories of being anxious. As adults, we still experience a lot of anxiety even though we have developed skills to control things. We still find ourselves worried, not about the supply of milk, but the steady and reliable source of income for ourselves and for the family we are forming. We may not be worried about the mother who may or may not return but we are concerned over finding someone to love us, or over our children's safety. Yes, we can manipulate the world as adults, but there are too many factors we cannot control and that makes us anxious.

But we have to emphasize still that anxiety is a legitimate and normal feeling. It may be a negative feeling because we are stressed by it, but it does not automatically mean that it is pathological. Anxiety is in fact very important because it makes us anticipate future actions, allowing us to prepare. You feel anxious about an incoming rain, so you bring an umbrella in case. You are anxious about the results of your grades, so you study very hard. You are anxious about a project proposal, so you spend sleepless night preparing for the presentation. We are anxious because the future event we are worried about means something to us. You can only be worried by something that you feel is important to you. For example, kids will not be excited that your company will be given a very big project. It might indirectly benefit them but it doesn't concern them so they aren't worried too much about it. If you are living in Africa, Thanksgiving Day might not be important to you because it is not your tradition and culture. You wouldn't worry about getting a turkey and inviting friends over. We can only be anxious about the things that are important to us.

Anxiety will only become pathological when we take it to the extreme of stressing ourselves too much and controlling everything. There is a normal threshold to anxiety, which allows us to be functional while worrying. But the pathological side of anxiety comes in when we try to control everything too much to the point that we become obsessed with the results. For example, if you have an upcoming bid for a project, it is normal for you to be anxious about whether you will get it or not. You might constantly be checking your email or your phone for any sign of a confirmation. If the waiting period is a week, you might feel very uneasy the whole week but you will proceed to doing other activities that are part of your regular routine. But anxiety becomes pathological when you are just obsessed with knowing the results that you check your phone and email every minute when you know the results are still in a week. It is not normal when you abandon all other activities because you don't have the results yet. The worry will always be there, but when it impedes your normal functions, then you have to consider whether you are overly anxious.

Anxiety also is a physiological phenomenon. There are biochemical changes in the body when we feel anxious. There are two autonomic systems in the body: the sympathetic and the parasympathetic systems. The first one is our 'fight or flight' mode and kicks in when we are threatened or stressed. The second one is our 'rest and digest' mode which takes care of the body and relaxes it, allowing for digestion to happen. They complement each other and control bodily functions. When we are anxious, the sympathetic system kicks in. This is primarily mediated by chemicals like epinephrine or adrenaline which signals the body that there is an incoming threat. Your heart starts beating faster, your blood vessels constrict, your metabolic processes become more active as you use up more energy and nutrients. The sympathetic system allows the body to respond to the threat whether it is real or imagined. It will kick in when you see a bus coming at you and will allow you to run faster than the usual. It will also kick in when you are watching a horror movie and you feel very tense. It is not real, but the body thinks the threat of a ghost is real so you sweat more and you feel more anxious. After the threat clears up, the parasympathetic system takes over to relax the body. Your heart slows down its beating, your vessels dilate, your breathing becomes deep and steady, your metabolism slows down.

When you become anxious all the time, the body will also have a lot of adrenaline in its system. It will always think that there is a threat that it needs to respond to, making you more tense all the time. This is not good because the parasympathetic system cannot do its job and you will simply feel tired and tensed all the time. If you have too much adrenaline, your heart rate increases and if this becomes frequent, it can precipitate a heart attack or some other cardiac event. Normal body function is altered because of the excess in chemicals, causing an imbalance which may cause diseases and damage structures in your body. The normal sympathetic and parasympathetic functions must be allowed to function at regular and equal intervals. The high levels of stress can trigger certain diseases like cancer or cardiopulmonary diseases if the anxiety is not controlled.

Cognitively, anxiety induces the person to think of the future in the present. Because it has not happened, you will think of scenarios that might happen. If you are going to present an important project, you will start thinking of possibilities. Maybe they won't like it, or you might stutter, or you might miss a slide. A question might be thrown at you which you might not be able to answer very well. If you allow your thoughts to run wild, they can even make connections which don't seem likely in the first place. From the anxiety of a project proposal, you might question your abilities and self-worth. Because you are anxious about your presentation, you might doubt your skills in speaking. The more you entertain these thoughts, the more they will become self-fulfilling prophecies that you are to blame for. You feel afraid because of the project, you doubt your abilities, so during the day itself, you stutter. It is a self-determining fear that paralyzes you, even though the event which you are afraid of has not transpired yet.

The brain is also not comfortable with waiting. If you are used to working a lot, then the sensory inputs will be over stimulated that it becomes very normal for you to do or think of something. These connections can go into haywire as the brain adapts to the frenzied activity. But, when there are occasions when the activity levels are low, your brain will feel strange and you will seek to return to your normal quick thinking on voluminous work. In reality, there are processes where you have no choice but to wait. When you are standing in line, you really have to wait for your queue. When you are expecting a baby, you really have to wait. If you are submitting a proposal, there is a window of waiting. And it is hard for us to accept that it is possible to do nothing when we wait for something. We cannot just sit and wait for an important event to happen to us.

And we ease the tension in a variety of ways. Anxiety can make people overly concerned about minor details. For example, when you were a kid, your parents were worried about your birthday party that on the day itself, they were still arranging the chairs, making sure that every last flower on the cake is perfect, every little balloon placed impeccably. These actions of nitpicking are a way of the body to release the tension.

But there are other possibilities aside from engaging in stressful anxiety-relieving activates. Instead of controlling the future all the time with our needless worrying, it might be good to approach anxiety through the two ways it manifests: physiological and cognitive.

Physiological alleviations of anxiety are designed to control the rush of adrenaline in our body. If there is really no threat in sight, the body should not feel too tenses. So you can apply breathing exercises to take in more air and nutrients. It might mean sleeping or resting, even eating. You can alleviate anxiety by drinking water or any non-caffeine containing products. You can induce relaxation by listening to peaceful music or taking a few moments to get some fresh air and enjoy the view. These will induce your physiological body to calm down and let the worry disappear.

Cognitive alleviations tend to look at the mental process in an anxious person and stop the train of thoughts. Usually, anxious people overthink things, so when you want to remove the stress, the first thing you do is to empty your mind. It could be simply sitting still and watching your environment, without conscious thinking. You will feel relaxed after just not thinking at all. Or you could be self-reflexive and ask yourself, "Is there anything I can really do to change the future?" If you have done your best, then the only thing is to allow the process to take place and wait for results. You can train your brain to focus on other things aside from the event you are anxious of. If you are waiting for the results of your exam which will be due in a week's time, you can try to get your mind off the exam by watching a movie, going out with friends or engage in your hobby. The more that you think about the results, the more anxious and stressed you will be. And the stress does not even change the results. You might be worried about a project proposal, but in the end, what does the worrying really do? Nothing. It only fills you with unnecessary negative feelings that make you more depressed or stressed.

The rest of the book will be your guide to relax more and feel the stress less. Remember that anxiety is normal because it alerts us to the things that are important to us. But it can also be pathological if we worry needlessly and unnecessarily, to the point of disregarding other important functions. There is only so much we can do in the present to prepare for the future. And we must learn to accept and practice the art of waiting. Hopefully, this book can help you realize and apply that in your life.

Chapter 7: Spirituality

PsychCentral.com (10) give whole host of reasons why spirituality is good for your stress levels. Some of them are very good reasons. If you believe in a higher power than yourself, you tend to be much more careful with your life. The page at Psych Central points to the work of Harold Koenig, M.D., associate professor of medicine and psychiatry at Duke University on stress management and spirituality. Being a spiritual person myself, I can explain this in another way. When you become spiritual, you learn that you and your opinion are not what the world revolves around. That sounds a little harsh, but you can actually stress about the color of lipstick that you wear, and if that isn't a plain enough sign that you need something more important in your life, then I don't know what is. Spiritual people don't stress over things such as this and see the world as offering opportunity rather than disaster.

So how do you embrace spirituality?

Many people associate spirituality with religion, though if you were to talk to some people about religion, you would find to your astonishment that they are not particularly spiritual. Spirituality comes from embracing life. It comes from appreciating what a small part you play in life and accepting something called "humility." A lot of people have a problem with humility and don't understand its connection with spirituality, but the difference between being religious and keeping to the rules you see as correct for your religion and being spiritual – actually becoming empathetic and humble in your beliefs – is huge.

Exercise in Spirituality

This is the most effective exercise that I can think of in spirituality because it puts you to the test. It makes you look at yourself honestly and when you do, you may be pleasantly surprised about what you find. If you live in a city, perhaps you don't see the sky very much. If you live in the country, perhaps what surrounds you is something that you take for granted. In this exercise you need to get beyond how you usually see things. Go to a place that you find to be awe inspiring but look at it in a different way. Instead of grabbing photographs or looking and then looking away at something else, really absorb what you see. I find the best time for this is sunset or sunrise. In yoga, we do an exercise which is called the Sun Salutation and that's something you can do at a later date to reinforce what you are expected to do in this exercise.

Look at the sight that you have chosen and feel the awe. One of the most important things that you need to see from this situation is how small you are in comparison with that beautiful scene. Why would you want to do this? It is something that needs to be acknowledged before you can embrace spirituality. You have to see yourself for what you are. You are one grain of sand on a whole beach. You are one pebble on the shore. You are a tiny speck of dust when it comes to how wonderful the world is. You are just a small atom compared to everything that you see.

How humility helps your stress levels

When you see yourself for what you really are, you also see life in a very different way. You begin to see purpose and sense to your life that you cannot possibly see until you get who you are in proportion. Humility helps stress levels because you are able to see everything more clearly. You learn to empathize which means that you are able to put yourself in other people's shoes. Thus, things that may have stressed you in the past are less likely to because you see things from the perspective of others as well as yourself. When you come this close to the reality of life, you also find that your spiritual beliefs become deeper and you are able to cope much better with what life throws at you.

How visualization works

This is another method that you can use to diminish your high stress levels. When things go wrong in life, you need a safe haven. Close your eyes for this exercise and think of a time and place within your life when things were happier. Imagine the scene, feel the emotions and you can use this as a safe haven for when things start to go wrong. If you find yourself stressing unnecessarily, you can take yourself to a quiet place away from negative influence and close your eyes and go to that safe place. This will give you space from the negativity of the situation and relax your mind, making you more capable of making decisions once you go back to the situation which caused the stress in the first place.

Take some time to choose your dream visualization because if you can think to a time in your life when you had no stress at all and everything associated with the memory is positive, this can help you so much to control stress, anger and all the negative effects that you may be experiencing in your life. Close your eyes and be there. This is your safe harbor.

Chapter 8: Psychological Self-Defense

There are many reasons why you would hold your tongue; these habits make you timid. If you are intimidated by others, you have little chance of standing up for yourself and your ideas.

You hold a set of boundaries which are intrinsically yours; if you habitually allow others to violate and otherwise overstep these boundaries, you put yourself in the position of less confidence.

You must work on 'self-defense' in various senses of the word to protect your psychological health. You need to be able to identify emotional leeches, defend your ideas in the intellectual square, and protect your body if you're ever attacked.

With this, you can feel true confidence about holding your true opinions, and feel assured that you can back them up if they're ever challenged.

Here's a brief list on how to do so.

- Physical: If you can't stand up for yourself, or realistically defend yourself from others, you might become intimidated.

So join a gym, and get into physical shape (cardio & weight-lifting) and learn to fight even if you don't want to start fights with others (MMA, boxing, Brazilian Ji-Jitzu).

- Mental: As bad as it is to not be able to defend yourself, it's doubly bad not to be able to defend your ideas from scrutiny.

Learn to structure your ideas logically; learn Aristotelian logic, even go so far as to read Aristotle's Organon (Categories, On Interpretation, Prior Analytics, Posterior Analytics, Topics, Sophistical Refutations).

Learn the Trivium (Grammar, Logic, Rhetoric); a great book by Sister Miriam Joseph. Take public speaking courses (Toastmasters has chapters all across the world). Get into dialectical debates with others (in which you're simply bouncing ideas informally).

Also, learn how to spot faulty logic (fallacies); this is where people find creative and deceptive ways of submitting bad logic. The worst part is that these ideas seem plausible, because they convince other people to betray their better judgment and to ascribe to bad ideas.

- Emotional: Fix your emotional dysfunctions, because several people in modern society are narcissists and sociopathic. Thus, they know how to leverage victim's emotions against them. Learn to recognize the signs of a manipulator. Recognize the injection of guilt, shame, and fear from others, and either cut away or call it out. This can be done with a quick Google search.

- Financial: The fear of loss of finances keeps many people from being fully self-confident. If you're concerned about the loss of finances due to your ideas, that might keep you from expressing yourself fully.

Either make the choice to accept the losses; make sure you have extra income on the side. Also, make sure that you find ways of generating income on your own, either via your own services, or passively over the web, so that you are not beholden to the work culture of self-censorship.

On an advanced level, financial dependence on others, even an employer, can stifle your confidence. You can start a side business, which can eventually provide full-time income to replace your current job.

Chapter 9: Managing Anger In A Healthy

Way

I have had so many clients ask me, "How do I stop feeling angry?" as if being angry is an unnatural emotion. It's certainly not. Most of us think of anger as some sort of a wild, negative emotion, and it's true to an extent. It not only makes you feel bad about yourself and others, but it compels you to do stupid things without realizing the repercussions your actions may cause. To avoid this, some "civilized people" start masking their anger or find a way to suppress it. Does it work? Of course not! When you suppress negative emotions, they are likely to come back with a vengeance and cause more damage in the long run than you expected.

Let us all understand that anger is a very natural human emotion, which can also have its upside if handled with care. You don't have to fight to make your anger go away – it's there for a reason. Instead of going against it, let's see how we can express anger in healthy ways whenever it arises so it sets us free.

Vent it out to a friend

Perhaps you are angry at a personal or professional situation, and it's making you anxious and vengeful. This is the perfect time to call up a friend and ask if he or she can spare some time and listen to you for a while. Catch up over a cup of coffee and really vent it out, even exaggerate the situation as much as you can. Tell your friend exactly how you feel, and how the situation is making you feel worried, helpless, anxious and betrayed. After you are done venting, thank your friend and let them know that you aren't expecting them to help with your situation and that you simply needed to vent. If your friend does come up with an opinion about the situation voluntarily, you may just have an AHA moment, and look at the situation from a different point of view. However, do not talk to your friend about the same situation again as constant venting can turn into recontamination very quickly which can be harmful for the body, mind, spirit or even the friendship.

Write a letter

Yes, this may seem funny, but it's one of the most effective techniques to get your feelings out. Grab a sheet of paper and address the letter to whoever may have been the cause of your anger, explaining how you feel. Once you dump your feelings out on the page, you can throw it away or burn it. This technique can help the anger stewing in our bodies find an outlet so it can stop rolling around in our consciousness. The clarity you get from writing down your thoughts can literally uproot all the negative emotions and give you a closure.

Scream

To scream or not to scream? I say go scream — just not at other people. But screaming your heart out in an open space, in your car or into a pillow can allow your anger to get a release. When someone ticks you off, you may want to react immediately to situation and may accidentally end up saying something you may regret later. You would rather hold off the anger, only to scream it off later and relive your frustration. Remember, that screaming and anger are not the same, and yet screaming can actually have a cathartic effect. For some, it can even prove to be extremely therapeutic.

Turn your anger into art

Allow yourself to go all Taylor Swift-y and pen down a song or just paint, come up with a poem, sing – use art to transform your anger. Just do anything that can count as creativity and watch your anger take your art to a different level altogether. It may be surprising, but anger can be a perfect muse. I have a friend who sketches out beautiful images on a canvas whenever she feels negative and trust me, some of her most powerful images came when she was feeling immense rage. The next time you feel like lashing out at someone, just immerse yourself in art and turn into something beautiful.

Talk to the person in a calm manner

If you can communicate your anger in a healthy way, you may actually start bettering your communication skills as a result. When someone is angry with you, or you are angry with someone, take a step back and give yourself some space from the situation. Maintaining emotional distance from the situation can bring you much clarity, and get you ready to talk to the concerned person in a calm manner. A word of caution: you will also have to be ready for some harsh feedback from the other person – so do this if and only when you feel emotionally ready.

Chapter 10: Ways To Improve Self

Confidence

While there are numerous reasons for low self-confidence, it is generally not productive to play the blame game. Parents are the usual targets, but it's important to remember that they did their best. Exploring the steps we can take to improve self-confidence is a much better use of time and energy.

Most of us have experienced or will experience some degree of low self-confidence at some point in our lifetime. If you have ever been the victim of job loss, your self-confidence has probably been shaken or, in some cases, totally shattered. Why me? I guess I just didn't measure up! These are negative thoughts and counter-productive. To restore or improve self-confidence, you will need to acknowledge the problem and proceed with determination to take positive steps to resolve the problem. Self-confidence affects every area of your life. If you are unemployed or under-employed, strong healthy self-confidence is absolutely vital to your success. Although your self-confidence may have been affected by circumstances beyond your control (unemployment, for example), there are many proactive ways to improve self-confidence. Remember, self-confidence affects your mental, physical and emotional health and your investment of time and energy in self-improvement will be well spent. So, let's get started.

First of all, you must make the decision that you can change and then make the commitment to yourself that it starts today. A huge part of any change or improvement takes place in your mind. Taking control of your mind and the negative thoughts that often run wild is a giant step in the right direction. This means you will be doing a lot of self-talk as your self-confidence increases. This self-talk is also known as "positive affirmations". These affirmations can be verbal or silent but need to be repeated frequently, consistently and with emotion. For example: I am intelligent. I am capable. I feel positive and confident. With repetition and over time, these positive affirmations will sink into your subconscious mind and one day, you will really feel positive and confident.

Another action step you can take is preparation - always "be prepared". If you are employed, be sure you are prepared for the work day. Whether you have a big assignment due or a simple task, be sure you are prepared and ready to meet your deadlines. This will reduce stress at work and will improve your finished product whether it is a major presentation for the company or a simple memo. Preparation for your work and refusal to procrastinate will result in a great finished product. Knowing that you were ready for the assignment and completed the task to the best of your ability will result in personal pride and more self-confidence. It is important to strive to be a person of excellence. If you are unemployed, preparation for the job search and job interviews will reduce your stress and build your confidence. When you approach a job interview well prepared, the possibility of a successful outcome is significantly greater.

Another way to improve self-confidence is expanding your knowledge and improving your skills. Consider taking a class to learn more about a subject that interests you. This will improve your ability to engage in intelligent conversation with others and boost your self-confidence. If you need more training in a skill that affects your career, take a class or attend a seminar. As your skill level improves so does your self-confidence. The current job market demands employees with excellent skills that will be top performers and add value to the company.

As your self-confidence grows, you will find yourself handling stressful situations with a calm mind. Each time you successfully handle difficult situations (big or small), your self-confidence is strengthened. Your calmness enables you to think clearly and use your ability to successfully complete the task at hand. Over time, these small steps will provide the self-confidence you need to achieve goals, both professional and personal. You will feel positive about yourself and your life and will move forward with the expectation of total success. So, don't procrastinate; the sooner you begin to improve your self-confidence, the sooner you will enjoy more success in your life.

In order to get ahead in life, we need to have a healthy dose of self confidence. Very rarely will you find someone who is successful in life but has a terrible sense of self confidence. This is because in order to succeed you need to first believe in your own ability for success, otherwise you will never get ahead in life. The thing you need to remember is this: Even the most confident person would have, at some point in their life, wish that they could be more confident, because with confidence comes success. Here are 5 great tips on how you can improve self confidence.

The first thing you should do is to stop being negative. You know how it is, it always begins with some minor little flaw that you think you might have. It may be excess weight here, some facial imperfection there, and then before you know it you start hating yourself for the way you look, thinking that people must think of you as some hideous freak, which would explain why no one loves you.

Learn to love yourself for who you are. What others think of you is not nearly as important as what you think of yourself. If you constantly put yourself down then you will never be able to build a healthy sense of self confidence. Whenever you feel that negativity start creeping up on you, the best thing you can do for yourself is to banish it from your mind and focus on the positive.

Speaking of focusing on the positive, the next step you can consider is to focus on your strengths. This can mean anything from your talents to your positive traits. Expand on your talents by joining some hobby group where you can get the acknowledgment and recognition for your talents that you deserve, and this will go a long way in boosting your self confidence to phenomenal heights.

The third way you can build on your self confidence is to set for yourself some small goals or milestones. You may have some dream waiting for you in the horizon, but along the way it is good to have milestones which you can achieve in order to get a boost of self confidence as you trudge along towards your eventual big dream. Remember, visualize your big dream as a mountain, and your milestones would serve as checkpoints where you can stop and evaluate yourself as you pass each one in your journey ahead. The accomplishment of each milestone will serve as encouragement for you to keep working.

The fourth way you can improve self confidence is to remember your past achievements. Recall how great you felt when you last achieved some great event in your life. It doesn't quite matter when you might have achieved it. It could have something to do with your childhood, or perhaps it had happened when you got your first job. Focus on the happiness derived from the event, and you will find yourself craving to achieve that same sense of happiness and satisfaction, and this will serve as motivation for you to keep building your self confidence.

The last way for you to improve your confidence is to celebrate your failures. This may sound absurd to you initially, but think of your failures as milestones to success. To paraphrase a certain celebrity, you should always prepare for glory by failing until you don't. Success doesn't come overnight, so learn to see your failures as you getting one step closer to success. Each failure is just another way for you to learn a new, better approach of doing things.

Chapter 11: How To Become More

Outgoing

Below are the few steps that help you become an outgoing person:

Split it and then apply it.

For becoming more sociable and outgoing, you need to set gradual steps for being outgoing and take these steps one by one. For example, you can start by asking questions in group settings, and when you become comfortable with that, you can continue with making more statements in group settings.

In time, gradually you'll finally find yourself becoming a socializing, lean, and mean machine. In learning how to be more outgoing and social, it's crucial to understand that this gradual process is what works best and to stick to it devotedly.

Set your Standard

One feature of shy people is that they set lofty social standards for themselves. They demand of themselves to make a great first impression, to be liked by all, and they think that if it doesn't happen it's a failure.

The individuals, who have very high social skills, can't rise up to such idealistic standards either. For this reason, one of the best things you can do to become more outgoing is to set your own real standards. If your standard for success is to get everybody to like you, then you're bound to be timid. But if your standard is simply to have discussion with new people, then you're bound to be more sociable.

The important thing you may need to understand is that you don't have to demand that much of yourself socially. You're only human, you will connect well with some people, you won't connect with others at all, and that's absolutely Fine. Accept it and live your life.

Manage Your Self-Talk

People tend to set their social bar high through self talk. They say to themselves that "I must make an impression on this person, they must show liking for me" and other stuff like that. If you look at these self talks and analyze them, you will find that it's full of crap and are useless.

Thus, to be more outgoing and social, you should learn to manage your self-talk. This means identifying the brainless, impractical or dysfunctional things that you say to yourself and willingly making them correct. As you do this in a systematic way, not only your regular self-talk changes, but the underlying attitude change as well. This helps you to get confidence and interact with ease to other people.

As you become more sociable, your people skills increase and develop as well. This makes you even more friendly and sociable.

Ways to overcome Fear, stress and anxiety

1) Breathing exercise:

By controlling breathing, you control all anxiety symptoms. Therefore, if you begin to feel anxious:

-Pause

Concentrate on the breath

-You can take your breath in (to the fast count of 7 in your mind)

-Then gradually breathe out (to the quick count of 11 in your mind)

If you exercise this for a minute or so, you'll be surprised to see how quickly you've relaxed. This is called '7/11 breathing' however the numbers varies, just as the out-breath is longer than the in-breath.

2) Get ready for a peaceful performance

If you get nervous about any upcoming activity or event, you notice that just thinking about that conference, speech, or interview or whatever will start to create physical responses – called anxiety.

Therefore, when you discover yourself imagining about some events which is going to happen in future, act 7/11 breathing. One of the symptom of excess fear or anxiety is not able to think clearly but in majority of modern places we want to keep clear thought.

3) Get control on your thoughts

Fear and nervousness increase when we think of the worst. People develop imagination to project the future; as a result they can plan in advance. Some people exploit their thoughts continually and so experience much more nervousness than those who fruitfully future-project their thoughts for those who don't think about the future at all. Nervous, constant worried people tend to exploit their thoughts to the extent that future events feel like disasters. No doubt their whole lives may be ruined by panic and nervousness.

4) Don't take the view point of others to your heart.

For happy and satisfying life, you need to be able to genuinely do things that bring happiness and joy to you. Often the view points and decisions of others hampers your authenticity. You should not allow this to happen in your lives.

No matter what people do, assume, feel, or say, don't take it personally. If they tell you that you are wonderful, they are not saying that because of you. You know that you are wonderful. It is not essential to believe other people who tell you that you are wonderful. Don't take anything personally.

5) Don't be hesitant to ask for help.

The enthusiasm and the guts to face a problem mean recognizing and talking about the problem, looking at the resources available at hand, recognizing solutions and options, and developing an action plan that will work the best.

Asking for help is a symbol of maturity and not flaw. It is an important part in developing an action plan. A lot of times we cannot see things clearly while facing the problem. Seeking for help can show us unusual ways of dealing a problem that we may have never thought of ourselves—there is always something to be learned.

6) Meditation

Meditation significantly reduces anxiety, stress and tension levels. Mindful meditation reinforces a person's thinking ability to control emotions." The ability to control our emotions helps us in dealing with our stress in a much improved way. Meditation has also helped in making the person relax and calm.

7) Be tolerant and patient.

Whenever you have a feeling of intolerant and restlessness, try to remind yourself that you need to embrace present living instead of wanting to be at another place than where you currently are.

The present is the only time that has purpose and meaning right now. When we become impatient and rush through life, we are probably missing out on important lessons and are deprived of full benefits of life.

8) Avoid comparison with others.

This might sound difficult, but we need to keep in mind that we are unique individuals; we should not compare ourselves with others. Comparing ourselves to others will only result in low self esteem and increase the stress and anxiety level.

9) Take the help of a therapist.

Try to find someone who you can speak to you in a confidential, secure place without any judgments. It is a totally outside perspective that may result in transparency and insight.

10) Do self care

Watch your favorite movie. Take a bubble bath.Go for a Spa. The options are unlimited, but the idea is to pamper yourself and relax. At times, it is necessary to just take care of yourself.

Chapter 12: Dynamic Duo: Diet & Exercise

Jimmy's daily routine had been the same for 10 years, rarely any variation. He would rise at 6am, shower, get dressed, hop in the car for his morning ride to work. On the way, he would stop at a fast food restaurant and consume a couple muffin, egg, cheese, and sausage sandwiches and head to work. He works for 4 or 5 hours and has his compulsory lunch of more fast food followed by a big, thick milkshake. He'd work for a few hours more, head home and when he arrived, he would order a pizza, take out Chinese, or cook some frozen burritos in the microwave. If he really wanted to splurge, he'd hit the local all-you-can-eat buffet. He began having panic attacks when he tried to cook at home, causing him to be immobilized until he went out somewhere to eat. His health continued to decline until he was overcome with anxiety and couldn't bring himself to leave his cramped little apartment.

Jimmy's story, while tragic, is an object lesson in how a sedentary lifestyle coupled with a diet of processed foods can change and ruin an individual's life. Poor eating habits have been linked to type II diabetes (which can greatly impact moods and emotional stability), coronary disease, pulmonary dysfunction, liver disease, gastrointestinal problems, and in some cases poor diet can bring about an untimely death.

Likewise, a sedentary lifestyle can bring about increased stress, obesity, muscle tissue degeneration, pulmonary distress, coronary disease, and a plethora of internal injuries. The easiest way to tell if a sedentary lifestyle has become problematic, is when trying to walk a flight of stairs, or carry groceries for a distance. If you become out of breath or unnecessarily tired, the affects of a lazy lifestyle have begun to hit - and that, in and of itself, increases stress and anxiety.

Exercise and diet are considered the "dynamic duo" where a healthy mind and body are concerned. When you combine a healthy diet with consistent exercise, the aggregate result is amazing synergy and a reduction in stressors that may have brought about the anxiety to begin with.

Here are a few tips for diet and then exercise that anyone can use and to a person, these tips will help reduce stress levels, anxiety, and panic attacks.

Diet

1.No Fried Foods: Fried foods are everywhere and they are simply horrible for a human body. Eliminating fried, battered foods must be the first stop on the improved diet train.

2.Timing:It's true what they say about eating after 9pm - don't do it. Your body is going into relaxation mode at that time of day, and intake of calories at that hour does not turn into anything but fat. So, do not eat after 9pm.

3.Fresh Is Good. Whenever possible, fresh, locally grown fruits and vegetables are the preferred choice. They aren't hard to find, if you're serious about fresh foods. Even the national grocery chains have a section of their produce that is "organically grown."

4.More Fruits & Vegetables: Organically-grown, locally produced fruits and vegetables are packed with nutrients and for good measure, supports the local economy. Think about it this way - when you are preparing a plate, make sure that half of the space on the place is filled with fruits and vegetables.

5.Honey Bee: At your local farmer's market and even some locally-owned grocery stores, you can purchase honey that was made from local bees. The benefits are two-fold. First, you'll be able to satisfy those cravings for something sweet with a teaspoon of delicious honey drizzled over scrambled eggs, tortillas, or perhaps your low-carb pancakes. Second, there are viruses and bacteria in the air that are unique to your region, the place where you choose to live. Local honey contains vitamins and protects against local allergies, and it contains antioxidants that the body needs on a regular basis. It acts as a sort of vaccine against localized, pollen related allergies.

6.Lean Protein: Your body needs proteins on a daily basis for physical and mental health. Whenever possible, the safe bet is to choose a lean protein. This is not to say, of course, you need to adopt a completely vegetarian diet, but it is important to note that many legumes are a great source of proteins. When purchasing meat, look for the leanest cuts, the easiest to remove the fat from, and then, avoid the temptation to load it up with sauces.

7.Lower Sodium: If you read labels, you will find that next to high fructose corn syrup saturation, sodium content is pervasive in every canned or prepared foods. Reducing sodium levels in one's diet will reduce the risk of coronary obstructions, and weight will be lost almost immediately. When you begin to see the impact that simply reducing your sodium can have on your body, the mind follows suit and becomes more confident, less prone to anxiety.

8.Reduced Sugars:"High fructose corn syrup" may sound healthy because, after all, the word "corn" is included in the name, but it truly is not. The amount of high fructose corn syrup found in most processed foods and sweets has increased exponentially in western culture and because it is cheap to produce and highly effective, companies will continue to use it as a sweetener. And the more it's used, the fatter and more sluggish we become. The physical impact translates into emotional problems because the mind doesn't slow down, but the body's ability to keep up is dramatically changed.

9.Water Is Life: Our bodies are comprised mostly of water, but clean, fresh water is something we seem to lack. For men, consumption of water should at least be 13 cups. For women, about 9 cups per day. That is most likely far different from what your actual intake might be.Water provides nourishment, hydration which is good for the digestive system, and gets the metabolism kicking.

10.No Soda: Soft drinks, even the "sugar free" options are just about the worst thing you could ever put into your body. Not only is the sugar/high fructose corn syrup off the charts, but the diet sodas contain aspartame which has been directly linked to many physical ailments. The jolt received from soft drinks, sodas, is only temporary and departs quickly, leaving the body craving more for that fresh jolt. Avoid sodas at all costs.

Those diet tips are all designed to provide you with healthy alternatives for your diet that isn't packed with depression-causing or anxiety producing chemicals. By changing your diet even slightly, you'll see a dramatic change quickly. And as you maintain a more healthy diet, the effects will be long term.

Exercise

1.Habit-Forming:When you begin any exercise routine, you'll find that it becomes addictive, and habit-forming. The body in motion causes the brain to produce endorphins that bring about pleasure and peace. The more you get regular exercise, the better your body will feel and when that happens, you experience less anxiety, and a lowered probability of panic attacks.

2.Start Small: If you're starting from the place of a completely sedentary life, a simple walk around the block is a great place to start. If you have been moderately exercising, it's time to start from the beginning and make it a regular occurance, a scheduled part of your day (see above).

3.Set Goals: Forget about weight loss and consciously trying to attack anxiety and your panic attacks. Concentrate only on the accomplishment of exercise itself. If you walk around the block, set a goal of walking four times around the block. Set goals that are realistic, yet obtainable. Track your results, write them down, and celebrate when you exceed your expectations.

4.Stick to Basics: Cardio is the primary resource when exercising to improve health. Producing some sweat should be the goal, not amassing muscles that would make Arnold jealous. A simple, basic cardio routine beginning with twice a week and leading up to every day is exactly what will help you overcome anxiety and even some of your panic attacks.

First, we have reminded ourselves that we're not alone in this struggle. Second, you have learned to identify your triggers and the circumstances that bring about your anxiety and possible panic attacks. Third, we considered alternative supplements to help you handle anxiety naturally and without pharmaceuticals. Fourth, we just learned how diet and exercise can be the "dynamic duo" in the fight against anxiety and panic attacks.

Chapter 13: Social Anxiety Support

Sometimes, it may not be you but a friend who is suffering from social anxiety disorder. Being in a supportive environment or having a friend, who they can talk to, often helps the person recover faster. You need to maintain a great amount of patience in order to help them get through the process of recovery.

•Stop encouraging anxiety behaviors: If you have a close friend or a family member who has been long suffering from this disorder, you may have developed certain habit to avoid their anxiety provoking situations.

•Suggest treatment: You friend may be reluctant to go seek help and even refuse to believe that there is a problem. Gently encourage them to get medical help as try explaining how the disorder is impacting their growth in life.

•Appreciate the smallest achievements: Remember it's a delicate period when your friend is trying to recover. It is important to recognize the efforts of the person by making them feel that you are indeed proud of them.

•Be patient: Recovery from social anxiety is a slow process and you need to be patient with them. It's a pattern build over the years and will take more time to break. Do not lay too many expectations on them too soon.

•Be a good listener: Just having somebody who can listen to their problems can relieve the stress they feel. You might feel that their problems are petty and illogical; however it may be extremely troublesome for them.

•Manage your own emotions: It's natural for a person with social anxiety to feel panicky or anxious in some situations. Do not get too carried away with their emotions and hold yourself. Try to be empathetic towards them but do not focus on the fear factor.

•Do not blame: Don't try to blame the friend every time they fail to control their emotions. They may be trying their best but due to habit they might not be able to control their behaviors at times

•Ask them what they need: Do not assume that you know what they need. If they find themselves in a socially anxious situation, ask them what it is that you can do to help them cope.

Chapter 14: How To Develop The Habit Of

Mindfulness

Mindfulness is easier said than done. Developing mindfulness is a way of building something good in your life so that you don't forget about living in the present. In order to develop a habit of mindfulness, you need triggers so that you can be reminded to come back to awareness when your mind wanders. Triggers help to make your daily activities become meditative thus making them a lifetime habit.

Mindfulness triggers can range from post-it notes on your computer or kitchen wall to mentally attached triggers. Mentally attached triggers are actions that involve changing from doing one thing to another. Consider mindful trigger very powerful 'wake up calls'.

The triggers are supposed to help you avoid your 'auto pilot'. You need to choose a particular event that reminds you to be mindful when it occurs. For instance, when you set a phone ringing as a trigger, you can choose to focus your attention on the sensation of breath to interrupt the process of reaction when it rings. This will give you a moment to step back. Giving yourself a little distance can help you experience the emotions in your body without fueling them but simply focusing on the trigger.

Another trigger worth noticing is when checking on your watch to see what time it is. Use this time to take a few deep breaths and notice any anxiety or stress that is making you check on your time. Allow the tension to settle before changing to another activity or going back to what you were originally doing.

You can set a trigger for when you are drinking water, when you walk through a doorway, when you turn on a light switch, while surfing the web, brushing or waiting anywhere for anything. Pay attention to the physical sensation present in the body or mental states present in the mind at that very moment.

After being mindful of physical sensation, expand your awareness to improve your current overall mood. Include your awareness to the presence of any thoughts at that particular moment. This way, you are becoming mindful again and again throughout the day. This form of practice will give your formal practice a great boost while making it more efficient.

This kind of informal meditation is an excellent way to get the most out of whatever formal meditation time you might have.

Although there isn't a right and wrong way to be mindful, some things you might do could prevent you from experiencing the benefits you expect so much from mindfulness. To ensure that you don't end up making it difficult for yourself to experience the full power of being mindful, here are some common mistakes to avoid.

Common Mindfulness Mistakes To Avoid

Expecting a particular outcome

You should not practice a specific mindfulness exercise expecting any certain outcome. Also, don't expect that the particular exercise will make you feel relaxed. You don't practice meditation to get better at the mindfulness. You practice mindfulness to wake up. You might feel relaxed or not. What matters is being in the present.

Trying too hard

Don't make things more complicated than they need to be. You can set your intention to bring your awareness to the present moment regardless of what happens next.

Waiting for the perfect moment

There are no perfect conditions for practicing mindfulness. It is ok to practice mindfulness informally anywhere you feel comfortable. In fact, informal mindfulness practice is quite more powerful in increasing compassion for you. Practice makes perfect. Therefore, don't wait for that perfect moment because every little bit helps.

Getting hijacked

Getting back your attention to your breath while practicing mindfulness is a beautiful way to focus your mind. This is not as easy as it sounds. It is not long before we are hijacked by our thoughts and emotions. This is a very normal behavior of our brain and it does not mean that you are doing anything wrong.

When you notice the thoughts, do not judge them; simply acknowledge them and let them pass. Be gentle on yourself and start again.

Forgetting

Our busy lives have made forgetting things a common part of our life and mindfulness is no exception to this. Put a reminder somewhere you can easily notice it to always remind you to be mindful. Commit yourself to practicing mindfulness by reviewing its benefits. The use of the triggers we mentioned above is a great way to unplug from the autopilot mode.

Sleeping during the exercise

Chances of you sleeping are very high if you meditate right after a meal, especially if you are a beginner. It is important that you stay inwardly alert while practicing mindfulness. To achieve this, try meditating early in the morning when you wake up. Second, you are likely to have better results if you meditate some hours after a meal. Third, sit upright in a cross-legged pose if you're the kind to meditate while lying down. Finally, do not meditate while under the influence of drugs or alcohol. If you are serious about meditation, avoid the use of such because it makes you less sensitive to the subtle sensory experience of mindfulness.

Finding mindfulness too religious

It all depends on the approach you follow. The exercises described above are non-secular and can be practiced by someone of any faith. Once you review the benefits, you will have no time for judgment whether they are religious or not.

Boredom

Dealing with boredom is a big problem in mindfulness practice. Boredom is associated with lack of enthusiasm and connection. Being bored shows lack of mindfulness. It means that you are dwelling so much on the past or the future.

To deal with it, acknowledge the feeling and accept the moment, notice the thoughts that are running in your head, and then get interested in boredom. Allow yourself to become curious like where is it coming from and where is it going?

Connect your attention to the sensation of breathing, and then take a step back from the emotion of boredom. You will notice that being aware of boredom loosens the feeling and lets go.

Overthinking

Overthinking during meditation traps us in a mental loop, which is hard to disengage.

Negative overthinking makes you feel trapped in your mind. Repetitive negative thoughts can lead to anxiety, stress, and clinical depression. It is hard to meditate in the middle of an overthinking episode but it is a tool to help you tame your mind.

While practicing mindfulness as a beginner, you might feel like you are giving your thoughts a chance to flourish. Simply acknowledge the thoughts and slowly return your attention to breathing for five minutes. This will teach your brain to have control, calm and relax for long.

Chapter 15: Things That Can Trigger

Anxiety Disorder

Everyone gets restless, frazzled, and anxious-but once you start experiencing constant anxiety and can't trace it to anything, you could have anxiety disorder. Doctors make diagnosis of generalized anxiety disorder when patients have anxiety symptoms like difficulty concentrating , frequent headaches, and constant worry for over six months without any good reason. Though the causes of anxiety disorders are not known yet, but certain triggers of anxiety disorders have been identified such as thyroid problems and weight-loss supplements.

Heart Problems

If you have ever had a panic attack, it means you are quite familiar with how your hands can get moist, you can't catch your breath-and your heart feels like it will pound right out of your chest. But most anxieties can be caused by problems with your heart. Most people after they have gone through some heart-surgeries and heart attack experience some anxiety symptoms such as shortness of breath and palpitation. These symptoms can last up to a year or more, and mostly occur in women.

•Alcohol and drugs

People with anxiety disorders, especially social anxiety disorders are about three times more likely to have issues with drugs and alcohol. But that is not all: Alcohol and drugs abuse can equally lead to anxiety disorder and an anxiety attack. People suffering social anxiety who abuse alcohol have been found to have serious anxiety symptoms-as well as several other emotional problems and health conditions. No matter what problem comes first, a combination of alcohol, drugs, and anxiety can form a very vicious cycle.

•Caffeine

Caffeine is a very powerful stimulant and can be a very bad thing for someone suffering anxiety disorder. In fact, the effect of caffeine on your body can be likened to a very frightening event. This is because caffeine stimulates your fight or fright response, and researches have shown that this can worsen your anxiety attacks. And just like the known symptoms of anxiety, the intake of several cups of coffee can leave you feeling moody, nervous, and awake all through the night.

• Medications

Certain medications come with very ugly side effects-they can cause severe anxiety symptoms or even trigger an anxiety attack. Prescriptions to be careful with include asthma drugs, thyroid drugs, over the counter decongestants and combination cold remedies can put at risk. And if you suddenly stop taking drugs to control your anxiety symptoms, the sudden withdrawal can cause anxiety symptoms.

Weight Loss Supplements

Most over-the-counter weight loss supplements come with anxiety-producing side effects. Saint John's wort side effects may include insomnia, and green tea extracts (which claim to suppress appetite) contain lots of caffeine.

Your Thyroid Gland

Your thyroid gland is a butterfly-shaped gland in the front of your neck that produces thyroid hormones. This hormone is very important for the regulation of your metabolism and energy levels. But if your thyroid produces lots of hormones, it can lead to anxiety symptoms, such as irritability, heart palpitations, nervousness, and sleeplessness.If you notice anxiety symptoms coupled with weight loss, swelling in the neck, fatigue, heat intolerance,

orweakness

, you need to have your thyroid gland checked by your doctor.

Stress

Stress and anxiety are known to go hand in hand. Stress is known to result in serious anxiety symptoms, and anxiety can worsen the stress. When you are very tense, you may equally resort to other behaviors that make anxiety worse such as drug abuse, smoking, or alcohol abuse. Don't forget that anxiety and stress are often accompanied by physical symptoms such as headache, stomachache, dizziness, dry mouth, and sweating. If you have symptoms of anxiety whose origin cannot be traced, you need to talk to your doctor. It is important to note that all anxiety disorders are quite treatable.

Chapter 16: Coping Strategies

Learning to live a productive life, able to interact meaningfully with others, is important to all of us.Any one of us is on a scale from having absolutely no problems (highly unlikely) to being totally debilitated by it.We can all learn something about our social relationships and should perhaps view it as a constant learning curve.

We will never be able to rid ourselves of anxiety completely but we can adopt strategies for dealing with it and recognize our own useless ways of dealing with things.Which ones of the following do you think you could incorporate to improve your coping behavior?

Flight/Fight/Freeze – Our body uses this mechanism to help us avoid or escape danger and has been passed down through the millennia to help us escape real danger. Our bodies have adapted this response to help us deal with problems in current situations. For instance, we might freeze when we are called upon to speak in front of a group. Or we might take offence and start a fight when someone criticizes us, even if it has been intended constructively. Or we might just turn round and take flight instead of going into the restaurant to meet our new date. We must learn to moderate this alarm and try and push ourselves out of our comfort zone; become aware of when we are using this strategy and try and walk through it.

Avoidance – You probably know that the longer you put off a task you find a little disconcerting, the harder it becomes to tackle, until it actually becomes insurmountable. We then develop feelings of guilt for not having tackled it.For example, you have been meaning to join a group but cannot pluck up the courage to go so you keep making up excuses to yourself – and others. You feel disappointed with yourself and start giving yourself negative talk: I'm not interesting enough/It's too far/I will feel silly. Face your worries. Take little steps. The first task is to show up!Sit down. Say hello.

Break things down. And then practice. It will get easier and before you know it, you will be enjoying yourself.

Deep Breathing – Practice this. Breathe from your diaphragm. Slow your breathing down. Babies use this and it is used in yoga. It is impossible to feel anxious when you are breathing slowly and become aware of it. It is easier to notice maybe the reverse, that when you feel anxious or panicky your breath becomes sharp and short and you might even hyperventilate. If you learn to take deep breaths when you feel a trigger setting off, it will help you to ride out the panic attack and bring your anxiety levels down. The saying, 'Take a deep breath' really does have some truth in it.

Progressive Muscle Relaxation – this is often used in meditation. You can start at the toes and tense them for ten seconds and then relax them. Work up your body: calves; knees; thighs etc. This helps to relieve overall stress and can also help with physical ailments such as headaches.

You should aim to do this exercise for around ten minutes, in a quiet place where you won't be disturbed. The more accomplished you become at this exercise, the quicker it will take effect. Use some calming music if it helps.

Helpful Thinking – Trying to second-guess what others are thinking of you is pointless. 'They will think I am fat/stupid/boring. 'What is the point of trying to guess what others are thinking about you? It is just that: a guess. You are bound to be harder on yourself than others. You might want to be a size 0 or just generally more attractive but others might already think you're gorgeous. It's only you who are expecting such high achievements of yourself. What would you tell your friend if she said she thought everyone considered her to be ugly/daft/boring?

Self-Awareness – You should become aware of exactly what it is that you are afraid of and write it down. Ask yourself if your fears are rational? Are they based on fact? If not, get rid of those fears. Are they helping you? What's the worst that could happen if your fears come true? Everyone does something stupid at some time. Try and develop a sense of humor and this should encompass being able to laugh at yourself too. Normally, when you become aware of your fears, you are more able to face them and evaluation makes it clear that they have no substance.

Write things down – Write down one of your fears, it helps us to be more logical if we see it in black and white. Write down an experience you know you would normally feel anxious about. For example, let's say you are going to meet a new friend at a restaurant. What fears would you normally have? What to wear? Would you look out of place? Everyone would look at me. The person I want to be friends with will not turn up. They will stare at me when I eat or drink and think I am disgusting. And then force yourself to question what has happened to make you think like this. Is it based on fact? Or are these irrational fears? You get back from the restaurant. Return to your list. What happened? So you noticed your jacket was showing its label. Did they call the police? Did everyone turn to stare? You are only guessing. It is fiction, not fact. Everyone makes mistakes and no-one is perfect.

As you start along this journey, you might develop some of your own techniques which you find useful. Use them as often and regularly as you need to.

Chapter 17: Depression Cure: A Healthy

Diet

"Let food be thy medicine, thy medicine shall be thy food." (Hippocrates)

Have you ever noticed feeling tired and bloated after eating highly processed foods rich in simple carbs, sodium, saturated and trans fats, and sugar? Some examples would be potato chips, soda, and greasy hotdog sandwiches.

On the other hand, have you ever experienced feeling energized and happy after eating nutritious, organic, whole foods such as nuts, milk, fruits and vegetables?

The choice of food that you consume has a major impact on your mood levels. In fact, changing your diet is one of the most natural ways to cure depression. There are certain foods that you can incorporate into your daily meals to boost the effects of your overall depression treatment.

Foods that Help Cure Depression Naturally

This is a list of foods that are known to help reduce stress and combat depression:

Green, Leafy Vegetables. All the green, leafy vegetables are chock full of essential nutrients that support our body's growth, repair and resistance against diseases. These nutrients are in the form of vitamins, minerals, protein, unsaturated (good) fat, and complex carbohydrates. Instead of eating unhealthy simple carbs (such as white pasta, white bread or white rice) with your meal, why not substitute it with leafy greens instead? Some suggestions are spinach, kale, collards, cabbage, and lettuce. Steam them for a minute, season them with a bit of salt and you are good to go!

Foods Rich in Antioxidants. Depression is sometimes triggered by aging and bodily dysfunctions caused by damaging molecules referred to as "free radicals."

These are produced by our own body and can also be found in the environment. The brain is most susceptible to the damage caused by free radicals. The only way to combat this is by consuming foods rich in antioxidants.

Beta-carotene is an antioxidant and it can be found in yellow to orange tinged fruit and vegetables such as carrots, pumpkin, squash, apricots, cantaloupe, and sweet potato. Many leafy greens and vegetables also have beta-carotene (such as collards, spinach and broccoli) even if they do not have the yellow orange color.

Vitamin C is another highly potent antioxidant. It is also water soluble, which means that it is never stored in the body. This is why you need to consume the recommended amount of this vitamin everyday. You can get it from citrus fruits such as oranges, grapefruit and lemons, as well as in peppers, blueberries, kiwi, strawberries and tomatoes.

Vitamin E is another important antioxidant that you can find in vegetable oils, wheat germ, nuts and seeds.

Green tea is a beverage that all depressed patients are recommended to have everyday (but always make sure to ask your doctor about it). It is rich in catechins and flavonoids, which are disease-fighting antioxidants that are said to be even more powerful than vitamin C and E.

Complex Carbohydrates. Carbohydrate is a nutrient that our brain naturally craves for. Some studies have shown that eating carbs boosts the production of the brain chemical called "serotonin", which is responsible for keeping us happy.

Unfortunately, simple carbs make us unhealthy and will actually cause the mood levels to fluctuate. Instead, opt for complex carbs. These are the whole grains that are healthier and more satisfying.

Simple carbs are your cookies, cakes and white bread and pasta which would initially spike up serotonin levels and then shortly after cause it to dip and leaving you feeling depressed again. Complex carbs are more difficult to digest, therefore enabling a gradual and steady release of carbs into the bloodstream and keeping the serotonin levels regulated.

Lean Protein. Protein-rich foods that have low fat content such as tuna, eggs, lean beef (grass fed), mackerel, salmon, chicken and turkey contain the amino acid named "tyrosine". Research has shown that it can help boost the brain chemicals called dopamine and norepinephrine, which are responsible for keeping us alert and focused. Aside from meat, you can also get protein from peas, soy, yogurt, milk, and beans.

Foods Rich in Omega-3. Foods that are rich in omega-3 fatty acids are scientifically proven to improve mood. Research has even shown a direct link between omega-3 deficiency and depression. People who eat a small amount of omega-3 reflected higher rates of major depressive disorder compared to people who eat a lot of foods rich in omega-3. You can get your daily dose of omega-3 fatty acids from fatty fish such as sardines, anchovy, salmon, tuna, and mackerel. Flaxseed and nuts, soybean oil, and dark green leafy vegetables are also rich in omega-3.

Another option to get your daily dose of Omega-3 is to take fish oil capsules at 3,000 mg per day.

Foods with Vitamin D

Research has proven that those who do not have enough vitamin D are more likely to develop or exhibit symptoms of depression. It is an essential vitamin for the proper functioning of the neurological system and it also helps alleviate inflammation. Foods that are naturally rich in vitamin D are cod liver oil, various types of fish (such as herring, salmon, sardines), fortified cereals, dairy products and soy products (such as tofu and soy milk), oysters, caviar, sausages, ham and salami, eggs and mushrooms.

Selenium-rich Food

This very important micronutrient can help boost the brain and combat depression due to its high level of antioxidants called glutathione peroxidase. This helps prevent the polyunsaturated acids in our cell membranes from becoming oxidized. It has also been reported that it boosts mood levels. You can obtain selenium from nuts, grains, oysters, and organ meats.

Overall, a healthy, balanced diet that is composed mostly of organic whole foods will make you feel healthier and happier. In contrast, there are certain foods that you should avoid or consume at a minimum in order to help cure your depression.

Foods that Promote Depression (and you should avoid):

Here is a list of foods that you should stay away from in order to cure depression:

Aspartame. This is an artificial sweetener that can put anyone at risk for developing depression. It inhibits the production of serotonin and causes insomnia, headaches and an overall bad mood.

Refined Sugar. While candy bars can give you that "sugar rush" or that surge of energy, this will last for only 20 minutes, causing your blood glucose level to dip drastically and leaving you with a disrupted mood and low energy once more. Constantly eating foods high in refined sugar are also linked to sleep disorders.

Highly Processed Food. If you are suffering from depression, try to avoid anything that has been processed in a factory. These foods are high in all of the bad stuff (simple carbs, artificial sweeteners, trans fats, preservatives, and so on) that cause fatigue, anxiety, irritation and depression.

Hydrogenated Oil. Trans fats are found in hydrogenated oil, and many fried foods such as fried chicken and French fries contain a lot of this. Even cakes and cookies contain it. Trans fats can clog arteries and restrict blood flow to the brain and a wide array of diseases, including mood disorders such as depression.

Sodium-rich foods. Too much sodium will cause an imbalance in the neurological system and trigger depression. It can also cause fatigue due to its negative effects on the immune system. Furthermore, sodium is the main cause of bloating and fluid retention. Avoid eating packed noodles and salty foods.

Caffeine. Anxiety and depression can be triggered even by small amount of caffeine. It disrupts sleep and affects mood. It also triggers nervousness and overexcitement. Avoid energy drinks, especially, as they contain 14 times the amount of caffeine in soda.

Alcohol. Avoid alcohol at all costs because it is a widely known depressant. It causes the central nervous system to malfunction which affects your thought processes, including your ability to reason and think. Drinking alcohol can also have a direct effect on your mood and make your existing depressive state worse.

You can also find out which foods affect your mood the most by keeping a food diary. For 20 to 30 days, take a picture of all the foods that you eat or write them down in a notebook. At the end of the day you can write down how you felt that day, and describe your mood in detail. You will be able to identify the food and beverages that usually trigger your depressive state based on your notes.

Chapter 18: The Future And & More Help

There is an overriding aspect of childhood that has a direct effect on children and forms a part of virtually every day of their young lives.

The future.

We are in a position where our lives have begun to take shape; we have a career, relationships, and our own home...basically we have a sense of who we are.

As a child none of this is mapped out for you and it's both exciting and worrying in equal measure, kids will have ups and downs just as we do in adulthood.

As parents we just have to do our best.

Part of doing our best is knowing our own limitations, It's also not unnatural for you feel overawed and there is nothing wrong with you asking for assistance or further advice from others including professionals who specialize in certain areas that your child has an issue in. It's not failing or admitting defeat, it's you getting the best you can for your child.

Some of the scenarios we've mentioned are not natural or comfortable to find yourself involved in so there is no shame or indignity in you asking for help from a specialist in the relevant area.

Oftentimes we are actually too close and emotionally involved to make the best overall decision, ask for help if you need it and be assured that you have support available.

Chapter 19: Breathing Meditation

The very first thing you need to do is put on clothing that you can be comfortable sitting in. This can be your favorite pajama pants or your workout clothes. It just doesn't matter. You can meditate anywhere that you are. For your first time, you might want to be at home. As you practice, you can branch out to other places as you are more comfortable doing so.

Now, get comfortable. Lie down, sit up, stand, you do what makes you feel good. You are not going to move for a few minutes so pick a position that won't leave you stiff when you stand up.

Take a deep breath. Focus on the way that the air flows through your nose. Feel the air fill your lungs. Concentrate on that feeling. Don't hold your breath. Breathe out through your mouth. Feel the rhythm as it begins to form. In and out in a steady pace.

What does the air feel like coming in your chest? Is it cool? Does it feel clean? How does your body feel when it is full of air? What does it feel like when you are exhaling? Be aware of how each breath feels. Get to know your body.

What does the air taste like around you? As you breathe in, notice all the flavors in the room. How do they make you feel? Think about simple emotions. Do not try to analyze anything that you feel. Just accept that is how you feel and keep going. Later on, once you reach a meditative state, you can go back and ask yourself why you feel that way.

What are the smells around you? Think about the air and how it would feel if you were in your favorite spot. How is that different from what you smell right now?

What are the sounds around you? Concentrate on your music. What color does it make your mind see? How do those sounds change as you breathe?

Finally, what do you see? What colors are surrounding you? Do you see any shapes? Concentrate and see if these colors and shapes change as you breathe.

You may want to try counting up until you reach that final stage of meditation. Counting gives your mind a something to focus on. Don't worry, as your consciousness ascends to that meditative state, your counting will soon fade into the background.

All you need to do is breathe steadily. This may take longer the first few times that you attempt it. Meditation for your brain is like exercise for your body. The more that you exercise, the better shape that your body is in. The more you meditate, the easier it is for your mind to reach this state of meditation.

What you do when you reach this state is completely up to you. You can write down your thoughts. You can draw out what is in your mind. Some people even make music. The entire point is for you to discover yourself.

When you are finished. You can count back from 100 to 1. Focus on each one of your body parts as you do, so that you know exactly how they feel. Focus on any muscle aches and relax them as you go. Soon you will feel refreshed and ready to go about your day.

If you are looking for a way to exercise your mind and your body, you should try some simple yoga moves. Many areas have classes that will allow you to receive instruction from someone who knows how to prevent you from overstretching or causing yourself problems. Remember, there is no wrong way to meditate, so don't be scared to go for it. Be patient with yourself as you learn the process. Before you know it you will be telling everyone why they should be meditating.

Using a Mantra

If you are not able to block out the thoughts that come into your mind, try a mantra. The one that most people know about is the Om mantra and you simply breathe in as normal but sing the Om on the outward breath. This quietens the mind a little and allows you to get rid of excess thoughts. This is always going to be useful to people who have minds that chatter!

Chapter 20: Changing Negative Thoughts

To Positive Ones

Everybody has negative thoughts, occasionally. However, they become a problem if they overwhelm your life. Intense negativity can make you miserable and instill feelings of failure in you. The opposite is true if we employ positive thoughts.

Not everybody was born an optimist. Thus, do not beat yourself down if your thoughts incline towards the negative side. Nevertheless, it is important to try cultivating a positive attitude. Research shows that having a positive attitude towards life and everything it throws your way has many benefits.

What can you do to reverse your way of thinking? Focusing on your thoughts will be a great start to nurture a positive outlook on life. Analyze your thoughts. For instance, if you experience a challenging situation, assess how you think about the occurrence.

Do you have a negative mono-talk with yourself? Understand whom you criticize in your mind in such situations. If you always think negatively, you will experience obstacles in your personal growth. Admitting that you have a problem is the first step towards achieving a positive thinking attitude.

Most people with a problem of negative thinking focus only on the undesirable aspects of particular circumstances. For example, if you had a rough day at work. You made a presentation and finalized a number of tasks, but forget to make an important call.

If you find yourself dwelling on that one failed attempt for an entire evening instead of focusing on other good things that you did, then you need to change.

Others go to self-blame. If you work in a department, let's say sales, and you end up blaming yourself for its failures, that might damage your psychological health. By taking such blames, you do harm to your self-esteem.

A positive attitude will not come overnight. You have to start small. Start by trading your negative thoughts with positive thoughts. Instead of counting your inabilities, place focus on the few things you can do very well. As time goes by, you will learn to appreciate your success and give less attention to your failures.

Positive thinking is not a substitute for reality. It is all about taking a proactive approach on life. Instead of feeling down, positive thinking enables you to handle life challenges through getting effective methods of resolving conflicts.

It will take time before you transform your negative thinking to positive thinking. However, it will be worth it at the end, you will see.

Chapter 21: How To Answer "What Is

Your

Greatest Weakness?"

Originally published on September 4, 2019 in Interview Prep,

On-demand Video Courses

It's the interview question every job candidate

dreads: "What is your greatest weakness?"

And there's been a lot of bad advice out there

telling candidates they should say things like,

"I'm too much of a perfectionist."

Or,

"I work too hard."

I call bullsh*t. And so does the interviewer who's heard the same canned answer from every other

candidate!

In fact, if you respond with anything like the above answers, you'll likely not be considered for the job.

Instead, your interviewers will think you're being dishonest with your answer. Then, they'll question your honesty for all your other answers.

You can't give a canned answer to this question.

And you also can't evade the question.

Why you can't evade the "What's your greatest weakness?" question.

I remember in my first professional job my supervisor Nicolette and I had to conduct interviews to fill a position similar to mine. She and I interviewed one candidate I will never forget.

When Nicolette asked the candidate what her greatest strength was she immediately had an answer. But when asked what her greatest weakness was, she feigned the inability to think of anything at all. It was as if she never expected this question.

The candidate kept staring down with her eyebrows furrowed like she was trying hard to think but couldn't come up with anything. She wouldn't give an answer and asked if she could pass on the question and come back to it later, probably thinking Nicolette would forget. She didn't.

When Nicolette later came back to the question, the candidate did the same thing. She sat silently with that "thinking hard" look on her face. Nicolette had no problem waiting through the awkward silence. It was like they were playing chicken to see who would speak first!

I don't think the candidate ever did answer the question. We eventually ran out of time and had to begin the next part of her interview, a presentation she had to give to the rest of the search committee.

I remember how frustrated Nicolette was with the candidate afterward. She said to me, "Everyone has weaknesses! She should've been able to answer the question with something!" This left a bad taste in Nicolette's mouth.

The candidate did some other things in her presentation which knocked her out of the running for the position, but her evasion of the question

"What is your greatest weakness?" was the beginning of the end for her.

How to appropriately answer "What's your greatest weakness?"

So if you can't avoid the question or give a BS answer to "What are your greatest weaknesses?," how do you answer it without putting yourself in a negative light?

There is a way! Here's how:

1. Understand why it's being asked

First, it's important to consider why the interviewer might ask this question. It's not always to try to trick you or to try to make you look bad.

Sometimes the employer needs to know what kind of support or training you might require when first hired.

2. Listen to the question

Second, listen to the question and answer it the way it's being asked. If the interviewers only ask for one weakness, only give one. If they ask for weakness ES (plural), then show you can follow directions, but only give two!

(Believe me, this is not the time to start making a laundry list of your negatives!)

3. Avoid canned answers

Third, do NOT give a canned answer like the ones above.

Just don't.

Ever!

4. Never negate your strengths

Fourth, do NOT give the same answer you gave for

the greatest strengths question. I actually see people doing this all the time. They'll begin their answer with, "Well sometimes my strength is my weakness because...BLAH, BLAH, BLAH."

The last thing you want to do is negate your strengths!

5. Never answer with a trait

Fifth, do NOT give a personality trait as your answer.

Why? Because traits are ingrained and are difficult to change.

Instead, give a skill since skills can easily be learned.

No one person possesses every skill, so you probably have a few examples to choose from, allowing you to answer honestly.

Just make sure it's not a skill heavily required for the job. Instead use one only slightly related to the job.

6. Follow up with a positive

Sixth, once you briefly give your answer, then follow up with a positive on how you're either trying to overcome your weakness or how you're able to compensate for it.

An example would be if you aren't good at Excel and you won't be required to use it much in the job.

Here's how you might word this:

"While I have experience in using MS Excel, I'm not as well-versed in the more advanced features of the program. Therefore, I'm currently taking an online tutorial to familiarize myself with Excel's advanced functions so I can use it more fully if necessary."

Always make sure whatever example you use for your answer is an honest one that doesn't have too negative of an impact on your candidacy for the job.

More interview help

There are other common interview questions just as challenging as the question, "What are your greatest weaknesses?" For example:

• Can you tell us about yourself? (This one is never as easy as you it sounds!)

• What are your greatest strengths? (There is also a method to answering this question you should know!)

• Can you tell me about a time when...?

• Why should we hire you?

• And tons more!

I teach you appropriate ways to answer each of these questions in my on-demand program Steps to

Acing the Interview and Reducing Your Interview

Anxiety.

The program also includes:

• Strategies to give you the confidence to overcome the fear and stress of interviewing.

• What you've been doing wrong in past interviews and how to correct it.

• The best and most productive way to prepare for your next interview.

• Questions YOU should ask in the interview.

• How to win the interview in each stage: before, during, and after.

I encourage you to check it out well in advance of any upcoming interviews so you'll have time to prepare the best possible answers and land the job offer!

Chapter 22: Getting Prepared

Getting started with mediation is the scariest part, but it will get easier as you go along. With mediation, practice truly does make perfect. Just keep in mind that mediation has nothing to do with religion or spirituality. It can, but it is not necessary. All you need to do is be present in yourself. You'll learn to train your mind to brings thoughts to the forefront and increase your awareness. You'll be able to examine your place in this world as well as who you are. This can help you to make life style changes if you feel they are necessary, making it easier to be who you want to be.

Preparing to meditate:

Preparation can be the hardest part. These simple steps to prepare will have you able to start the mediation process in minutes. There's no reason to stress out about if everything is perfect. Just go down the list, but remember that nothing will be perfect.

You shouldn't wait for perfection to start meditation. Just get everything as good as you can before you begin.

Step One: Create a goal. The first thing you need to do is figure your goal that you're trying to achieve through mediation as well as how much you want to meditate. It's best if you meditate at least once a day, but you'll need to set out a specific time and schedule to meditate at.

This will make sure that you don't have an excuse not to. If you ever do have to skip, then reschedule it for later that day. Do not skip a day because you need to create a habit that you will follow. Find a good reason to meditate. If you don't have anything in mind, then your goal should be to rid yourself of your stress and anxiety, allowing yourself to become more relaxed and at peace.

Step Two: Find a spot to meditate. You may feel more comfortable going outside or staying inside. When you're just beginning to meditate, then it's recommended that you try and stay indoors as much as possible because it lacks as many distractions that will make you frustrated when you're trying to learn a new skill. Meditation is a skill that will take practice.

You will want to have a clean, comfortable spot. There's no reason to meditate on the hard ground if you find that to be uncomfortable. There's not even a reason to sit in a certain position if you don't feel comfortable. If you put yourself through any level of discomfort, then you're more likely to not be able to concentrate, and concentration is the key.

Meditation is impossible without it. You'll also want the spot that you have picked out to be a quiet one. Distractions will break your focus, and so if you're doing it in a house, you'll want to make sure that no one disturbs you. Getting back into a meditative state once it's broken is quite hard, especially for a beginner.

Step Three: Choose your clothing carefully. It doesn't mean that you need a perfect outfit. When you're meditating for the first time, you'll want to have comfortable clothing for the same reason as why you'll want a quiet, clean space. No distractions. Don't have that skirt that feels like you're a little too big around the middle. Don't have jewelry that feels heavy or distracting. Change into workout clothes if you need to.

As you get better, you'll be able to tune out these distractions a little easier, and then you'll be able to wear whatever you like. Jewelry will usually clink. You will concentrate on discomfort if you're trying to pick out something fashionable, and even your shoes will make a difference. Shoes can distract you, and many beginners will actually take their shoes off when they're just learning to meditate for the first time.

Step Four: Choose the proper time to start meditating. There is no best time for meditation, since you can really meditate just about anywhere at any time, but when you're beginning some times are better than others. Meditating right before bed and right after waking up is always recommended. It'll help you to clear your thoughts and either end or begin your day. You are also much less likely to get interrupted. However, if this does not work for your schedule, then you'll want to instead clear a time in your schedule to meditate.

The most important thing is that you are not disturbed no matter when you choose to do it. Trial and error will tell you what will actually work best, but planning beforehand is recommended. If you have an erratic schedule, just make it your goal to find time to meditate whenever you can. Once every twenty four hours is usually best, but if you have to, it can be once every other day. Try to increase the frequency of your meditation as time goes on, especially if you want to reap the benefits that meditation has to offer.

Step Five: Determine the length of your mediation session before you actually begin. As a beginner, you won't want to meditate too long. It'll be hard to keep meditating for an hour. It's recommended that you start with five to ten minutes a day. After each week, then you can increase it. You can even do meditation sessions more than once a day, but make sure to keep each session to a reasonable time when you're just beginning so that you don't become discouraged. Sometimes you will not be able to meet your goals, but that is human as well. Do not ever allow yourself to talk down to yourself or become too frustrated.

Chapter 23: Specific Fears

Sometimes fear can take over our lives and stop us from doing what we want or need to do in order to improve and enjoy our lives. In addition to the program I would like to share with you this quick guide for dealing with the most common fears.

Eleanor Roosevelt said this about fear, "You gain strength, courage, and confidence by every experience in which you really stop to look fear in the face. You are able to say to yourself, "I lived through this horror. I can take the next thing that comes along.""

Year after year the list of the most common fears remains the same and if you suffer from fear of public speaking, flying or heights you are not alone. Fear of flying is in fact so common that 1 in 3 Americans suffer from some level of this fear.

Fears, like anxiety, are not rooted in an objective truth but are results of our irrational beliefs. This is why fear of public speaking ranks much higher than the fear of dying.

Below are quick guides that will reduce and eliminate fear from your life.

8.1. FEAR OF PUBLIC SPEAKING

Public speaking does not necessary mean standing on a podium and giving a speech. Public speaking comes in lots of different forms. Fear of public speaking may be standing in your way of achieving personal and professional goals.

Scott Adams shared these words of encouragement, "We do not always have an accurate view of our own potential. I think most people who are frightened of public speaking and can not imagine they might feel different as a result of training. Do not assume you know how much potential you have. Sometimes the only way to know what you can do is to test yourself."

You can remove this fear by following these 18 steps:

1.Be prepared - write your speech and think about details of your upcoming speech. Write a script that details everything from taking your position to walking away.

2.Practice - go over your speech and learn it. Do not try to learn it by hard. Prepare bullet points that will allow you to keep your speech on track.

3.Get into a flow - during your practice runs find a rhythm to your speech.

4.Focus on your breathing - coordinate your breathing with the rhythm of the speech. Use pauses that occur due to breathing as a tool to increase the impact of your speech.

5.Practice in front of the mirror - use a mirror to practice and improve your facial expressions, gestures, posture and movements.

6.Get to know your voice - during the speech you will be able to hear yourself and for most people hearing their own voice for the first time can be disorientating as it sounds nothing like you expect. Record your speech and listen to it. This will allow you to get used to the sound of your voice and to improve your speech.

7.Practice in front of people - ask someone you feel comfortable with to listen to your speech. This will build up your speaking experience and you will get valuable advice.

8.Practice some more - use any opportunity you get to speak in front of a group of people. If you have regular meetings at work with suggestions part, prepare and give a short speech with some sort of suggestion. To gain more practice you can join your local public speaking class.

9.Exercise before the speech - if you ever watched comedy specials or recordings of live concerts you must have noticed one thing all performers did before going on stage - they all did a small exercise. You can do few jumping jacks, have a walk or do other exercise. This will loosen you up and it will burn a bit of that excess energy.

10.Prepare notes - to keep you on track you should have cards with speech key point prepared or you can use presentation tools for this purpose. You might not look at your notes once during the speech but just the knowledge that you have them will give you piece of mind. Have them just in case.

11.Eliminate fear of failure - go through concerns you have and eliminate them. For instance, you may be concerned that audience will be bored by your speech. To challenge this worry you can point out to yourself that your speech has few very interesting facts and your audience is comprised of professionals who will benefit greatly from the information you are going to share with them.

12.Focus on your speech not the audience - focus on delivering speech and information you are sharing.

13.Be well informed about the subject - do an extensive research about the subject. Having this additional information allows you to speak with more certainty and will remove fear of additional questions.

14.Embrace the fear - this fear is what motivates you to practice one more time. Use this fear to improve and remember that even people who give hundreds of speeches still get this fear.

15.Staying out of focus - do not try to read reactions of the audience. Shift your gaze in a pattern which will have you looking at every part of the audience without focusing on any one person.

16.Water - have a sip of water before giving a speech and always have water available during the speech. You can even integrate taking a sip of water during the speech to give it more drama or to emphasize a point.

17.Enjoy this experience - all these people are listening to you and most of them look up to you because you are able to speak in front of all these people. Take pride in this.

18.Constantly improve - use your experience from previous speech to improve your next one.

8.2. FEAR OF FLYING

Fear of flying is an extremely common one. This can be blamed on media coverage and on the lack of understanding of how planes function. Here are some tips that will help you next time to reach your destination without a burden of an additional baggage of anxiety.

1.Get informed - part of this fear stems from the lack of understanding or misunderstanding of flying. Watch some documentaries to learn how planes, dispatch service and airports work to keep you safe. Learn about the extraordinary safety statistics of flying.

2.Create a detailed plan - for some people fear of flying starts with the airport entrance. No wonder as you have limited time to navigate this maze like structure.

Use airport floor map to get acquainted with the route you will take to your gate. Prepare your documents and keep them in an order you will need them. Arrive at a time which will allow you to arrive at your gate with some time to spare.

3.Understand processes - security checks and requirement to show your documents can feel intrusive and can act as anxiety triggers. Use relaxation techniques and understand that these procedures are designed to keep you and everyone else safe.

4.Explore your fear - try to pin point what false belief your fear is based on. This may result in a realization that none single aspect of flying actually scares you.

5.Visualization - day before the flight, go through your next day in your imagination. Start with the taxi picking you up and end up with exiting on your destination safe and sound.

6.Try virtual reality - use virtual reality device to play out the flight while still on the ground. The use of virtual reality for exposure therapy has been proven to be effective and very cost efficient.

7.Use breathing and muscle relaxation techniques - use techniques you learned in the second chapter to relax during the flight.

8.Enjoy this experience - get a seat next to the window so you can look outside. The view of earth from the birds eye view is astonishing, magnificent and can not be compared to anything else. It is truly humbling and will help you put everything in perspective.

Seeing how small we are will help you realize how insignificant are issues you bother yourself with.

Flying opens up the great big world that is waiting to be discovered by you.

8.3. FEAR OF HEIGHTS

Fear of heights can vary from a fluttering in the tummy, to a full on panic attack. Avoiding being exposed to heights is not an answer.

Here are seven tips that will help you get this fear under control:

1.Explore your fear - in many circumstances, the fear of falling from heights is completely unfounded. Examine what do you fear specifically.

2.Notice safety equipment - when you feel fear taking you over, apply breathing exercise and when initial fear has subsided tell yourself "look at all this safety equipment that protects me from falling." Notice barriers, rails and other equipment installed on the site to keep you safe.

3.Visualization - imagine being on the roof of a building or on the hill. Use virtual reality glasses to visit Empire State Building viewing deck and similar places.

4.Gradual exposure - in order to conquer my fear of heights I jumped with a parachute. If you feel that this is too drastic for you, start gradually. Start off by walking over to a window and looking down. Gradually increase height and decrease barriers.

5.Do not do it alone - open up about your fear to people you trust and employ their help to overcome this obstacle.

6.Use breathing exercise - if you feel that fear is overpowering you, stop and use breathing exercise to regain your composure.

7.Use thought restructuring - employ positive self-talk and questions to change your automatic response.

Chapter 24: Developing Your Meditative

Practice

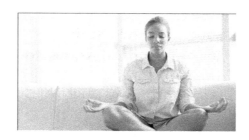

At this point we have taken some time discussing what meditation is, how it can benefit you and some of the many styles of meditation that are practiced worldwide today. A solid understanding of meditation is essential before you begin, but now you are probably wondering how exactly to get started and how to build a regular meditation routine.

Whichever method of meditation you choose, the ultimate goal is to become a quiet observer of your thoughts, allowing yourself to become detached enough to gain perspective on any situation and be able to see it through a balanced point of view. There are only four things that are absolutely essential to successful meditation.

Those things are:

• A quiet place to practice, be it solitary or in a group

• The ability to get yourself into a position where you breathe easily and maintain comfort for the duration of your meditation with as little movement as possible.

• If your meditation requires it, a focal point. This might be anything from an alter, the flickering flames of a single candle or an object that has significance that you consider soothing.

• Positivity and an open mind. Meditation can be difficult at first and you might feel discouraged. With the right attitude and an open mind you are practically guaranteed success.

If you are practicing meditation in your home, it is a nice idea to devote a specific space to your meditation, if possible. If you are short on space, maybe think of creating a meditation box or bag in which you keep your mat, pillow, focus object, music, guided meditations, meditation journal, or whatever objects help to make your meditation more successful and enjoyable. Treat it as a sacred space, one that is to remain untouched by stress and other negative emotions.

Although you don't necessarily have to stick with it, it is a good idea to decide on a time of day to practice meditation, at least to start. Eventually you will be able to practice meditation at any time that wish, but in the beginning practicing at the same time and place each day gives you the opportunity to become accustomed to the distractions that surround you, for example morning traffic outside your window or the chirping of crickets in the evening. When you become accustomed to these distractions it is easier to acknowledge them and regain your focus. This also is a good opportunity to learn how to observe from a distance. When you are able to remove yourself and place those distractions in the distance, you can begin to see them with renewed clarity. Soon, you will be able to approach other aspects of your life with the same type of distanced observation.

At this point, it is also important to mention that if you are suffering from depression and beginning meditation practice, that you might need to adjust your technique to serve you better. By this I mean that sometimes entering into mindfulness can feel isolating and a little scary if you are already plagued by feeling empty and alone. If you find this to be the case, take a step back and use your meditative time as a sacred time to focus on positivity. Following is a nice beginner meditation for positivity and balance. Unlike other meditations, you can use sensory inputs that bring you happiness.

Do you have a certain song that makes you feel centered or happy? Maybe you have a small token that reminds you of blessings that you would like to focus on or hold on to.

• Create an ambiance that brings you comfort and peace. Some ideas include incense, candles, a plush pillow, a blanket if you feel chilled, or an object to focus on that reminds you of happiness.

• Find a comfortable position where you can breathe freely and maintain your posture for at least ten to fifteen minutes. You can choose to sit up straight, or if you have had a particularly difficult day you might wish to recline of lay back on a soft surface.

• Close your eyes and breathe in to the count of ten. Fill your abdomen with your breath and breathe out, fully exhaling and emptying out your lungs.

• Now take another breath, but this time as you are breathing in, imagine the air around you being pink (or whatever color you associate with love and happiness). The air surrounds you and as you breathe in you will bring this love and happiness into your body.

• Let the pink air fill your body and feel it infuse every cell of your being. Concentrate on the feeling of this happiness spreading through your body from your head to your toes.

• As you breathe out, imagine a color that expresses negativity to you. You exhale the breath of this color and imagine it floating up and dissipating.

• Repeat this as many times as you needed to fill every bit of your body with the positive energy.

• Let your mind roam as it may, as long as the thoughts are pleasant in nature. If you find that your thoughts are turning towards negativity or the other things that fill your hectic life, breathe in more pink air and use it to erase the negativity from your mind.

• Once you are completely infused with positive energy, do one final breath and fully eliminate any negativity. Imagine yourself enveloped in a pink, protective bubble that surrounds you throughout your day.

• Once you are able to enter into mediation in a state of positivity you can then begin a mindfulness routine.

Use this time to focus on eliminating the negative thoughts from your mind and replacing them with positive ones. Continue on with this as long as you need to before you begin a more traditional meditation routine.

Chapter 25: Why Does My Body Go Into A

Panic Attack?

What is going on in the body during a panic attack? Why does this happen?

Feeling so frustrated and angry at my body for betraying me, was getting me nowhere fast. I would feel like I was on top of the anxiety and doing really well, then out of the blue a panic attack would hit and I would feel like I had been kicked to the ground. Most of the time it would take me a while to figure out why? I didn't understand what was happening to my body, I just knew I didn't like it and wanted it so badly to stop. I knew my mind was involved somehow but wasn't really sure how it related.

Knowledge is power, so it was time to find out.

Fear

Panic attacks are intense fear responses. They occur when there is no physical danger to the person that would usually trigger them. Instead, it is our thought processes that triggers them.

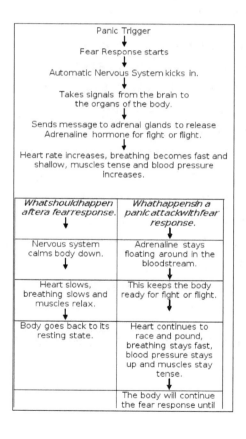

Panic Trigger
↓
Fear Response starts
↓
Automatic Nervous System kicks in.
↓
Takes signals from the brain to
the organs of the body.
↓
Sends message to adrenal glands to release
Adrenaline hormone for fight or flight.
↓
Heart rate increases, breathing becomes fast and
shallow, muscles tense and blood pressure
increases.

What should happen after a fear response.	What happens in a panic attack with fear response.
↓	↓
Nervous system calms body down. ↓	Adrenaline stays floating around in the bloodstream. ↓
Heart slows, breathing slows and muscles relax. ↓	This keeps the body ready for fight or flight. ↓
Body goes back to its resting state.	Heart continues to race and pound, breathing stays fast, blood pressure stays up and muscles stay tense. ↓
	The body will continue the fear response until

For those dealing with anxiety and panic attacks, the nervous system instead of calming the body down, continues to respond to the fear. This results in panic and anxiety.

Why does a person have the fear response resulting in anxiety and panic?

This will help explain your symptoms as you have a panic attack and the continued symptoms of anxiety. This knowledge is giving you the ability and tools to stand back and look at the anxiety and panic your body and brain are going through from the outside. This knowledge gives you the power to help you fight the fear response.

This fear response has evolved through time. In the beginning its purpose was to ready the body to protect it from danger.

Threat of physical danger from a vicious animal		
How Body Reacts	*Reason for reaction*	*How this relates to Panic attacks*
Sympathetic Nervous system kicks in Raises heart	This is for Fight or flight. Blood is needed fast at the large muscles like the	Feels like your heart is racing and is going to beat out of your chest. Sometimes can feel

rate Strengthens heart beat	thighs and biceps to get ready for action.	like a heart attack.
Blood is taken away from hands, fingers, feet and toes.	If injured the person will be less likely to bleed to death.	Feels like your hands are clammy and you have tingling sensations in your feet and toes.
Deep fast breathing.	This gets the tissues of the body more oxygen again in readiness for fight or flight.	Feels hard to breathe. Chest is tight, might even feel like you're being smothered. You could also feel dizzy and confused because blood to head is decreased by the heavy breathing.
Body produces more sweat.	Helps to stop the body from overheating while in action and makes the skin slippery and harder to grab if caught by the	Feel clammy and sweaty.

	animal.	
Brain changes focus of attention.	Need to be aware of what's around looking for danger.	This means that during a panic attack, you may have difficulty focusing on basic tasks, concentrating and your memory.

It takes time for everything in your body to settle back to some form of normal after a panic attack. With adrenaline still floating around in the blood stream your body is still charged up waiting for the fight or flight. It takes days for this adrenaline to be absorbed or used up. Remember the panic is a response to an unreasonable fear by your brain and body. It feels very real but you can combat it.

Move, Eat, Sleep, Do

In a panic attack your physical response and reactions feel out of control. Your body will often feel like you are running a marathon and as in a marathon you need to give your body the best chance at winning. To help you move through the panic, fight the anxiety and live requires that you move, eat and sleep.

Moving

Hard to do when you are in the middle of a panic attack but it is so important. Moving away from where you are having the panic attack can give your mind something to distract from the panic.

First step in the fight and taking control.

Moving in the form of exercise also helps the body release the excess adrenaline that is built up when you have a panic attack. It also helps the body release the feel good hormone to counteract the effects of the anxiety that you are often left with after a panic attack. Adrenaline will stay floating around in your blood stream being metabolized slowly unless you speed up the process by exercise.

Sleep

For me the thought of going to sleep on the days when panic attacks are happening or have happened is often enough to set off another one. The fear of being alone without anything to distract me is overpowering. Have a plan for what you are going to do on the nights of the panic.

To get to sleep on these highly anxious nights I do the following:

Read a book before I sleep. Then as I am trying to go to sleep I really focus on what the story was. The characters, the plot and anything else in the story that will keep my attention off myself.

Have a sleepy tea. Chamomile is known for its relaxing properties.

Take a Valerian or a blend of herbal sleep remedy.

Do the breathing exercises.

Sing a song in my head that I know the words to.

Usually the combination of these will get me to sleep. If you are having real trouble getting a good sleep and can't find a way that will work for you, then it's time to go see the Doc.

The goal is to give your body the best fighting chance of beating the panic attacks. You can't do this if you're not getting enough sleep, as sleep helps to reset the brain.

Eat

It seems that panic attacks keep coming on in waves. The first wave is so intense that you feel frozen. You fight through that, get moving and under control using your fight plan, then in the morning you wake up and its back again. Not quite as bad but still there. What do you do? How do you keep pushing through?

My last panic attack started at 10pm and had me frozen in my bed until 4am. Then I was wide awake at 6am able to get up but very confused and unable to focus easily or make decisions. The breathing and fight plan were working to keep me from leaving home and my family and running away. I was finding it really hard and felt terrified of it getting worse. I didn't want to 'snap' and not be responsible for me. This was the worst panic attack I have had in about a year. The fight plan had been working. But the fear and terror of it getting worse was making it worse.

At my worst, with my first ever panic attack, I was hospitalized and sedated. My mum came to look after me as I was incapable of getting out of bed. Each morning she would give me porridge to get me started. I knew I had to eat and because panic attacks make everything speed up, I knew it had to be good food that would last. I had forgotten, as you do when things are going great, that even eating when a panic attack lasts longer than a couple of hours is too much to think about. That it adds another layer to the panic to consider what to eat let alone what to feed anyone else.

I fell back on what mum fed me when I was at my worst. It worked then and having it already decided made me feel a little less freaked out.

Breakfast – Porridge, Not the packet stuff but the full rolled oats with sultanas and honey.

Lunch – Multigrain toast and eggs.

Dinner – Mashed potato, veggies and chicken.

Snacks – Fruit, slightly green bananas, Fruit and nut bars, dried fruit, Nuts or cut up veggies.

Why worry about eating when it's the last thing you feel like doing?

It is part of you owning the panic attack.

By eating you are giving your body a fighting chance. You can't run a marathon without having given your body good fuel to sustain it. This is the same with panic attacks. You need to replace the stores of energy you are using up while your body is in a state of panic.

I choose to give my body a fighting chance against this panic attack by feeding it good, sustaining food.

Remember your physical response and reactions may feel out of control when you're in panic mode. This makes it extra important to support your body through this. Eating good sustaining food helps your body keep up and feeds the fight to move through the panic.

Your turn:

List your go to meals/foods that you can fall back on while you are in panic mode. For me, my stomach is usually churning and I feel like throwing up. The foods I choose are pretty bland but filling and easy to throw together. See the next book – "Prepare your body for the fight!" for a more detailed look at foods that combat panic and anxiety.

Do

Distraction is a fantastic tool for combating panic. The plan is to distract your mind from the panic related thoughts by giving it something else to focus on. This can be anything that takes your full concentration.

Suduko

Crosswords

Find a words

Cooking

Coloring in

Craft

Sewing

Gardening

Keep it together

Remember it takes time for the adrenaline to be absorbed out of your blood stream. While it is floating around you will still feel the effects of the fight or flight response. The fear and panic feeling will stay in your body. Stay on the outside of it so you can look at it for what it is: an unreasonable fear reaction to an event or thought. The fact that you are reading this means you are giving yourself the tools and strategies to stop the fight before the first punch. Give yourself the best chance to rebuild slowly by keeping everything really simple for a week at least. Eat right, sleep well, nap when you need to, exercise and take away any stress. Cancel appointments, ask for help and keep that talk in your head all positive.

I've done it once.

I can do it again.

I have the knowledge and the tools

to heal quickly and get back to living.

Chapter 26: Tips To Reap The Benefits Of

Your Meditation

"Knowing is not enough; we must apply. Willing is not enough; we must do"

– Goethe -

–"Go slow; be gentle and compassionate with yourself." Catherine Kerr, Director of Translational NeuroScience at Brown University Contemplative Studies Initiative

–Make it a part of your daily routine. As you continuously practice meditation, you begin to enjoy the benefits.

–Always keep in mind your reason for meditating. There may come a time when you want to give up, don't! Remind yourself of your "why meditate."

–Keep at it. Meditation is not a one-time deal. Make it as much a part of your daily routine as brushing your teeth.

—Learn how to just be. You will benefit most by not analyzing the results of your daily practice. Just do what you can and let it go.

—You may find yourself becoming impatient, restless, even falling asleep; your mind may wander. Or you may experience real silence .... just go with it. Gently bring your attention back to your breathing whenever your awareness becomes sidetracked.

—In meditation, it is the act of focusing on what is important; in this technique it is the breath, not the distraction.

—When you close your eyes and focus on your breath, imagine how good that breath, that beautiful life-giving breath, makes you feel every time you inhale and exhale. Savor the beauty of those moments when you are completely aware of your breathing and nothing else. Don't question or form an opinion of what it means.

—Perfection is not the goal. If you try to be perfect, you missed the point of "just going with it."

—Relax. Let the magic happen and enjoy. Practicing meditation is a lifestyle. Some people may buy expensive cars, large homes and drape themselves in fine jewelry to impress others. You meditate to give yourself peace of mind, experience improved health, better relationships, and achieve greater happiness – that is impressive!

CPSIA information can be obtained
at www.ICGtesting.com
Printed in the USA
LVHW021029280720
661634LV00017B/777